ZEN MACROBIOTIC COOKING

Book of Oriental and Traditional Recipes

By MICHEL ABEHSERA

CITADEL PRESS   SECAUCUS, N.J.

TO MY FELLOW MAN—FOR
WHOM I WORRY AND DEDICATE
MY LIFE

Copyright © 1968 by Michael Abehsera.   All rights reserved.
Published by Citadel Press, a division of Lyle Stuart Inc.,
120 Enterprise Ave., Secaucus, N.J. 07094.   In Canada:
Musson Book Company, a division of General Publishing Co.
Limited, Don Mills, Ontario.   Manufactured in the United
States of America.   ISBN 0-8065-0893-0

Contents

Introduction   1
How the Author of This Book Became a Cook   7
A Simple Introduction to the Law of Opposites Before We Get to the Recipes   9
A Few Do's and Don'ts   12
Don't Worry About Essentials—They Are in Your Foods   15
The Vitamins   16
The Minerals   19
Recommendations   21
The Foods from Yang △ to Yin ▽   24
A Quick Summary of What You Will Learn   27
Before You Dive into Your Pots   32
Grains—Cereals   35
Rice, the King of Kings   35

Couscous   45
Crêpes and Pancakes   47
Millet   50
Breads   52
The Children of Grain   56
Secondary Foods   57
Nituke   57
Seaweed   65
Tempura   67
About Eating Only Rice   77
Hors d'oeuvres and Accompaniments   78
About Balance   91
Soups   93
About Fasting   126
Fish and Seafood   127
The Wisdom in Grains   147
"Main Dishes"   148
How About Cold Drinks?   161
Gomasio   162
Sesame Salt   162
About Chewing   163
The Worst Thing   164
Sauces   165
About Salt   171
Desserts   172
Little Things to Know   191
Bibliography   195
Monthly Publications   196
Glossary
Index

Introduction

Better is a dinner of herbs where love is, than a stalled ox and hatred therewith.

PROVERBS 15:17

Why is it called *Zen macrobiotic cooking?*

It *is,* basically, Zen cookery. It is the traditional food of ancient Japan, now preserved fully only in the Zen Buddhist monasteries. The rest of Japan, unfortunately, moves more and more away from this traditional cuisine as it becomes more and more like the West. Zen monks are the longest-lived and healthiest people in Japan while, at the other end of the scale, Westernized physicians and restaurant owners die early—these are the actual statistics in Japan, but they are ignored.

Zen monks, clinging to the ancient customs, cook and eat the foods described in this book. The term Zen macrobiotic was coined by Sakurazawa Nyoiti, better known in the Western world as George Ohsawa. He came to Zen cooking, not by tradition (he was raised as a Westernized Japanese), but in his search for health. He learned the scientifically sound principles underlying the ancient traditions. In bringing them, first to Westernized Japanese and then to movements which now flourish in all parts of the world, he had to find ways of teaching the ancient wisdom through words, phrases, new terms more readily comprehensible than much of the language of Zen.

One of the terms he coined is *macrobiotics*. It is derived from the Greek: *macro* means great, *bio* means vitality, and *biotics,* the techniques of rejuvenation.

Zen macrobiotic cooking, then, is the ancient Zen art of selecting and preparing food to produce longevity and rejuvenation, formulated in language suitable for people living today.

This book has as its aim to provide an easily understandable introduction to this kind of food selection and food preparation. If you know nothing about the Zen macrobiotic way of life—and this book is written on the assumption that it will be read by such newcomers—you can learn its art of food selection and preparation from this book and enjoy and benefit from such foods. No doubt you will be inspired to go on to read other books which will tell you much more about Zen macrobiotics as a way of life. Some of these books are listed in the bibliography at the end of this volume.

Even if you are altogether a newcomer to Zen macrobiotics, you already know about the essentials of this kind of food, if you stop to think for a moment.

Certainly you have known at one time or another that the staff of life to the Zen monks is rice, and you also will recall that the rice is not the polished white rice of modernity but the brown rice that you may even have seen in health food stores.

What you probably don't know is that the Zen monks were consummate chefs—only the most outstanding monks were allowed in the kitchen!—and made a dish for the gods out of rice.

You also probably know that the Zen monks were vegetarians. Zen macrobiotics is based on deep respect for this vegetarianism and follows it to a very considerable extent, but leaves room for fish and fowl as *secondary* foods. Unlike the traditional vegetarians, Zen macrobiotics considers fish—when part of a meal in which rice or other grains are primary, vegetables and fish secondary—a healthful food. Fowl is less healthful but, if organically fed, will do no harm. Zen macrobiotics agrees with vegetarians that beef and pork are unhealthful and dangerous, especially if eaten as a primary food. Meat finds its way into the Zen macrobiotic diet, quite simply, as a concession to man's sensual desires.

But this concession must be properly understood. First, it is a concession and only a concession. Second, if you wish seriously to enjoy the benefits of Zen macrobiotics, start out by cutting out meat altogether for as long as you can.

If you are in contact with students of Zen macrobiotics, you will hear them talking about the Number 7 Diet. This is a diet in which, usually for a period of ten days, one eats *only* rice. One then goes on to a series of graduated diets, identified as Number 5, Number 4, and so on, in which rice remains the prime food, but secondary foods are added.

The benefits of Zen macrobiotics can be thrown away very easily by overeating. The beginning of wisdom here is to stop overstuffing yourself, and even to stop stuffing yourself. Learn to stop eating before you are full. As a starter, get up from the table while you are still feeling a little hungry.

If you meet men and women who live the macrobiotic way of life, you will find them all, quite without exception, free from the American curse of overweight. This is not the result of calory-counting—there is no such thing in macrobiotics. It is the inevitable result of this method of food selection and food preparation.

Here is George Ohsawa's own simple and clear chart of diets or regimens (he preferred this word) to observe. One begins with Number 7, as I said, usually for ten days; one also goes back to Number 7 in case of illness. Numbers 6 to 3 should be where we spend most of our time. Those marked with minuses are slightly below the margin of safety, are resorted to occasionally in the search for variety, and are not recommended.

NO.	CEREALS	VEGS	SOUP	ANIMAL	FRUITS SALADS	DESSERT	DRINKING LIQUID
7	100%						Sparingly
6	90%	10%					"
5	80%	20%					"
4	70%	20%	10%				"
3	60%	30%	10%				"
2	50%	30%	10%	10%			"
1	40%	30%	10%	20%			"
-1	30%	30%	10%	20%	10%		"
-2	20%	30%	10%	25%	10%	5%	"
-3	10%	30%	10%	30%	15%	5%	"

* * *

Had I been asked five years ago to write a cookbook I would have been utterly amused, for I was in a precarious state of health and a cookbook for me was identified with a list of recipes for stuffing one's belly.

These five years have been an exhilarating adventure and happiness spent with a dear wife and children together with a "thousand" friends. The anguished thoughts of a 28-year-old have been dissipated and he has been freed from the tortures and agony that previously pervaded his existence.

This new and happy change has been due to the profound influence of George Ohsawa, who made it possible for me to recover my health so that I could leave France and journey to New York, the city of my dreams. Now, I have decided to write a cookbook. Not one for stuffing the belly but as a guide to health and to the exercise of better judgment in selecting foods that we should respectfully bring to our most cherished possession, our body.

Since, unfortunately, so many of my fellow men and women today suffer because of their stomachs, I approach you from the kitchen and introduce you to a new world of foods that are healthful, nourishing, and also delicious.

The true art of cooking is not one of subjective throwing together different combinations of food products combined with all sorts of fancy condiments to produce exotic flavors. It is judicious balancing of selected nutrients which produce nourishment as well as taste sensation. This is a great art which has been either forgotten or distorted through artificialities introduced into the menu of contemporary man.

Please, for the sake of your and your children's well-being, allow me to take you into this wonderful forgotten world of true natural body and spirit enchantment.

* * *

George Ohsawa was a man, a kind of magician, yes, who moved the mountain into the sea by the marriage of philosophy and cuisine. He came to us and, with the glee of the child of truth, said, look, life is nothing if not the meeting of opposites;

but the joyous unity, in skillful balance, of these opposites—therein lies the secret of life. In balance is harmony, beauty; in oneness, peace and the power to move mountains with a breath.

So went the gist of his philosophy and, if he wooed us, if he won us over with a certain undeniable passion, like a temptress, like a titillating Sophia flashing bare ankles above the slow and sensual dance of her feet, with jeweled bracelets of grandiose utopian promise, he did not leave us with that hopeless onanistic sterility of philosophical thought which dances divorced from life—no. He told us that from foods we are given life, and in the skillful joining and balancing of foods are we given the secret of life.

Such a simple statement, yet what shock of recognition whipped itself through our addled brains. We said, yes, maybe the answer to the riddle is so simple that we did not even dare try to find the voice, let alone muster the style, the weight and wit of argument, to embody it, to make it real to us and to the world. And here was this man telling us about the secret of life with all the headlong, unabashed simplicity of a child.

Yes, he won us over, and we practiced his philosophy and did not find it wanting.

* * *

I am deeply grateful to many of my dear friends among whom are David Grunes, John Bellicchi, Gloria Neil, Cecile Levin and Nina Zedicoff who assisted me in, first of all clarifying my French-oriented English jargon into acceptable English. If I have omitted anyone, I hope he will bear with me for this unpardonable lapse of memory. However, I must assure him that he is more firmly embedded in my heart, so mere acknowledgement hardly suffices to render my gratitude.

How the author of this book became a cook

It was a Saturday night when I decided to become a cook: Tell me, how much water do you use for that amount of noodles? Half a gallon, she said. She would be terse. Cooking was her last stronghold.

Well, do you have to boil the water first?

Yes, she answered, amused as if from a great distance, suddenly confident in the inviolability of her position. It takes a very long time to become a cook, she told me, as if I were a child.

* * *

On the following Monday evening, between 6 and 7 P.M., forty people appeared at the flat, congregating in the tiny living room in anticipation of the promised feast. Invitations had been sent three days in advance, telling of a private restaurant to be made out of our humble living quarters.

That same day, at 10 A.M., I had not even mastered the minor art of cooking an egg. I was terrified. My wife herself, frankly, was beginning to panic at the thought of the night ahead.

The meal, when it was finally served, was incredibly beautiful to look at—not to minimize its palatability; indeed, it all seemed the work of a master. I was the most amazed. How did I do it? I asked my wife. She gave me the usual story of how I am a genius and an incomparable husband, etc. My vanity blossomed—my cooking improved. It was the first time in my life that I found vanity to be extremely useful. Every day for eight months I experimented with a new dish. Then one day I found I had become a cook—or rather become recognized as one.

A simple introduction to the law of opposites before we get to the recipes

You don't have to understand this chapter to enjoy and profit from this recipe book. Just, please, read it and get from it what you can before going on to the recipes.

In Japan it is known as yin and yang. Here, in America, it goes by the rather chemical terms of acidity and alkalinity. For instance, you eat something acid and have heartburn; common knowledge tells you to take something alkaline, Alka-Seltzer, perhaps. Acid foods are rich in potassium; alkaline, in sodium.

We can equate it thus:

Yin = Acidity = Potassium = Sugar = Fruits, etc.
Yang = Alkalinity = Sodium = Salt = Cereals, etc.

Yin expands: sugar is yin. Sugar, when placed on the tongue, tends to make it expand.

Yang contracts: salt is yang. Salt, when placed on the tongue, tends to make it contract.

If any element affects the mouth, it invariably affects the body, which in turn affects the mind. What are commonly known as drugs can be taken generally as an extreme example of yin. Drugs, extremely acid, expand the mind, diffuse concentration, cloud sensibility, etc. Excessive eating and drinking by a longer yet equally efficient process bring about the same results. Yet do not be misled into thinking that acidity is bad! Acidity and alkalinity are necessary complementary opposites, good or bad in direct relation to quantity and balance.

In food, the perfect balance of alkalinity and acidity is found in only one grain—brown rice. Experts such as Dr. Rene Dubos, the Nobel prizewinner, tell us that we can possibly live on this cereal alone. It contains a balance of 5 parts potassium (yin) to 1 part sodium (yang). Thus, in eating other foods, it seems that if we adhere to this ratio of 5 to 1, we are in good hands.

If we eat rice exclusively, we need not worry about balancing it with other foods. Rice contains all the elements our bodies need. However, if we eat only meat, which is yang, we are not able to live in good health; a balance is necessary—some vegetables or some fruits. In a word, something yin. Even buckwheat, one of the yang cereals, must also be balanced by something yin, such as vegetables. We must keep balancing our meals or at least try to be as close as possible to the proper ratio. This kept in mind, there is yet another factor that enters the scene: our own individual need.

The 5-to-1 ratio may work for one person and not for another. A person who has much more potassium in his body surely needs more sodium; he would have to carefully introduce more sodium into his food, remembering, of course, that extreme action leads to extreme reaction.

Our cells, our body and mind keep changing all the time. Necessarily, our meals should follow this same law of change. What we are today we will not be tomorrow. Consequently, our meal of today should not be the same as the one of tomorrow. A very banal image of balance is the scale of justice. But there is another much more exciting image, that of the dynamic. We must modify our diet to fit with season and geography, time and place. Seasonal change is a drama in which we and our diet change also.

There is a proverb that says: Tell me with whom you associate and I will tell you who you are. This saying applies, not only to people, but also to our food. A man who eats only pork comes to resemble a pig and to behave like a pig in any circumstance. A meat eater is not as quiet as a vegetable eater. The meat eater gets angry easily. He is explosive, while the vegetable eater lives in the diurnal tranquility of a flower, opening to light, then closing with the day's end. A woman, if it is her wish to do so, can change the character of her husband by feeding him a certain kind of food. Choose your life! Wild or wise! Both perhaps, why not? Your destiny is on your tongue.

A few do's and don'ts

Learn above all to cook rice and to cook it well. One condition is to use a heavy cast-iron pot. Prior to cooking, wash the rice with cold water in a strainer. While cooking, never stir the rice, and keep it covered.

Don't make too much gomasio* in advance. It must not last more than a week or two. Close the container hermetically.

The best tea is made in teapots previously washed with boiled water. Leaves must never be boiled. However, roots and twigs must be boiled for a few minutes.

Avoid cooking foods over a high flame. Usually, unless I say otherwise, the flame should be high only at the beginning, until the boiling point.

---

* Terms marked with an asterisk throughout are explained in the Glossary at the end of this book and are also dealt with in later chapters.

Introduction « *13*

Don't throw away the green parts of vegetables such as carrots, radishes, etc. They may be used for soup.

Don't boil your vegetables. By sautéing rather than boiling them, you preserve valuable vitamins and minerals.

A nituke* should be almost dry; otherwise it will be like soup.

Add salt just before the end of your cooking; avoid adding it at the table.

The amount of salt varies according to the quality and the quantity of the food. A vegetable rich in potassium would require more sodium (salt, soya sauce, miso), although it is not a general rule. Some people may need this extra potassium.

Watch your intake of salt. Much salt brings about great thirst.

The best tempura* is made with oil heated to 350°F. constantly.

Stir your preparations with a wooden spoon or chopsticks. Metal spoons not only may damage your pots, but will "break" your vegetables while stirring or mixing.

It is better to cook with spring or well water. It is healthier and tastier.

Avoid cooking your foods in aluminum utensils. Clay, glass and cast-iron pots are preferable. Clay especially heightens the taste. Stainless steel is also recommended.

Vegetables should not be peeled. A special brush* (tawashi) is recommended for washing them. Rinse them under running water.

Sometimes when you cook rice, the bottom of the pot is slightly scorched. This part is yang. It is very rich in minerals and very good for yin people.

Avoid eating while you are cooking. Doing so may spoil your

ability to create. An empty stomach is one of the secrets of any creative activity.

A good Japanese knife, wide and heavy, is recommended for cutting vegetables. Work on a clean cutting board which should be washed as often as possible.

Don't worry about essentials—they are in your foods

Rice, always remember, is the best and most balanced cereal. That is why it is the principal food in this diet. When I say rice, I always mean brown rice. It should be served at every meal.

Oats are the grain richest in fat. *Corn* is the second richest. Again, *oats* are the richest in mineral salt; *barley* is next. *Oats, buckwheat* and *whole wheat* are the richest in protein. *Buckwheat* is the richest in magnesium, calcium and amino acids; its protein more than equals the best animal protein.

The vitamins

The discovery of vitamins is fairly recent. Vitamins were not a subject of conversation in the era of our grandparents; today they are a serious and daily preoccupation of families and business.

The consumption of vitamins today is due to an increase in population and a decrease of arable land, and very much due to the lack of organic fertilizers and the heedless commercialization of the food industry.

At the beginning of the 20th century, Casimir Funk demonstrated that brown rice contained in its first layer a substance able to cure beri-beri. Analysis showed the substance to be nitrogen in large quantity. From this discovery came the word *vitamin: vita = life, amine = amin = nitrogen = vitamin*.

VITAMIN A

Vitamins enable the tissues to resist contagious sicknesses. Vitamin A is in all vegetables, especially in those which have green leaves. *Parsley* is the richest: 30,000 International Units; *carrots*, 21,000; *dandelions*, 12,000; *lettuce*, 4,000; *pumpkin*, 2,500; *watercress*, 4,000; *escarole*, 15,000; *spinach*, 25,000. *Radish leaf, cabbage, cauliflower, wheat* and *chick peas* also contain vitamin A.

VITAMIN B

This most complex of all vitamins is divided into many categories. We shall consider four of them: B_1, B_2, B_6 and B_{12}.

Introduction « 17

B1: In the outer layer of rice. We find it in large quantity in *wheat germ* (yin), *yeast* (yin), in *whole wheat bread, rye, lentils, chick peas, chestnuts, nuts, egg yolk, raisins, cabbage, radish, dandelion* and *parsley*.

B2: In almost all the foods mentioned above. Also in all *cereals. Buckwheat* contains an enormous quantity of it.

B6: In all *cereals*.

B12: The most mysterious of all. Our need of this vitamin is small. We find it in the intestinal flora.

VITAMIN C

The lack of this vitamin is the cause of many deficiencies and very often of such serious diseases as scurvy. Captain Cook observed that while some animals such as sheep, goats, pigs and monkeys developed scurvy, others like rats, cats, dogs and birds did not. That is because the latter produce enough vitamins that they need from substances they find in their foods.

Vitamin C maintains the good structure of the body. Without it the blood vessels become porous; the muscles weak, sometimes weak enough to create paralysis; the mineral salts do not work effectively; anemia is general.

Vitamin C is destroyed by heat. However this does not apply in the case of brown rice. Recent work of Japanese and English scientists shows the existence in the covering of rice and other cereals of a pro-vitamin C resistant to 150° Centigrade heat and from which our bodies synthesize vitamin C.

Vitamin C is found in large quantity in *parsley, green cabbage, lettuce, onion,* the *green* of the *scallion, watercress, carrot tops, dandelion, radish leaf, strawberries* and the *skin* of the *apple*.

VITAMIN D

The Egyptians and the Chinese used to cure certain diseases by leaving the patient exposed to the sun. Today, it is well recognized that the sun is a benefactor; it gives to the body the opportunity to produce its own vitamin D.

Vitamin D is partly responsible for calcium metabolism; it is necessary for calcium absorption. It increases the amount of calcium in the blood and has the big responsibility of carrying it to the bones. This does not mean that the entire work is done by it alone; magnesium and phosphorous are two important elements which also help in this metabolism.

To cure rickets one needs vitamin D, calcium and phosphorous. Rickets occur either from a lack of calcium in our food or from a lack of vitamin D. Vitamin D and calcium are complementary and indispensable to each other. One helps the other to be well absorbed.

Vitamin D is found in the *sun,* all *cereals,* mostly in *oats, vegetables, oil, sardines* and *chicken.*

VITAMIN E

This is found in *rice,* all *whole cereals, vegetables, lettuce, watercress, olives* and in great quantity in *buckwheat.*

VITAMIN F

Vegetable oils, olives, olive oil and *sesame oil* contain vitamin F.

VITAMIN K

This is found in *cabbage, parsley, spinach, brown rice, carrot tops.* It is also produced by the intestinal flora.

The minerals

CALCIUM

Without calcium, blood cannot coagulate properly. Calcium deficiency creates hemorrhages, cramps, demineralization of bones among elderly people.

Too active parathyroid glands may rob calcium from the bones.

If you worry about, and need, calcium, you can find it in *watercress, dandelion, cabbage, carrot tops, parsley, seaweed, lentils, chestnuts* and in small quantity in *all cereals*.

PHOSPHOROUS

This needed mineral is in *all cereals, miso, soya sauce, parsley* and *lentils*.

MAGNESIUM

Found in *sea salt, all cereals* and *cabbage*.

IRON

Parsley, watercress, dandelion, carrots, scallions, lentils, soya, nuts and *all cereals* contain iron.

IODINE

This is found in *seaweed, agar-agar, watercress, all garden vegetables, fish*.

PROTEIN

All cereals and *vegetables, miso*, soy sauce*, sesame seeds* contain protein.

FAT

In *all vegetable oils* and *cereals*.

SUGAR

Found in *all cereals* (most in rice), *raisins, carrots, apples, lentils, nuts*.

---
* See glossary at end of book if you don't know any of these starred words.

Recommendations

In our very simple introduction to the law of opposites, I told you about yin and yang. You may see in the next pages the verbs "yangize" and "yinnize." To yangize is to produce constriction. This operation consists of *decreasing* the amount of yin elements, such as liquid, gas, potassium and other elements that exist in great quantities in the majority of vegetables and fruits. To yinnize, then, means the contrary: this consists of increasing the amount of yin elements.

According to the law of change you would eat yang in a cold (yin) climate: that means you would eat buckwheat, fish, all grains and vegetables such as burdock, carrots, etc. In a hot yang climate you would eat slightly more yin: vegetables and some fruits. However, no matter what the climate, you should always eat rice to stabilize your diet.

Always and everywhere avoid industrialized food and drink,

such as sugar, soft drinks, dyed foods, all canned and bottled foods, etc.

Also avoid any fruits and vegetables artificially grown with chemical fertilizers and/or insecticides.

If you have a preference for spicy foods, use those with the subtlest flavor; they are less harmful to the body, especially the stomach.

Try not to eat any food that is grown far away and in a climate contrary to your own.

Try to avoid any vegetable or fruit out of season.

Eliminate completely from your diet the most yin vegetables: potatoes, tomatoes and eggplant. These three vegetables are extremely high in potassium and have been known to be poisonous to the body when consumed in excess. In fact, it is told that the Incas used eggplant and tomatoes to induce susceptibility to illnesses such as syphilis in the Spaniards, their conquerors.

Eliminate coffee.

Eliminate teas containing carcinogen dye. This means practically all the teas in the usual packages.

Most animal foods and their byproducts are chemically treated and thus should be avoided. This means you should eat only organic meats and fowl. Wild birds, fresh fish and shellfish are preferred.

Avoid drinking while you eat.

A golden rule: drink after meals; not too hot, not too cold and by little sips. This last advice is recommended for those who complain of indigestion and stomach aches.

Good chewing is an important factor of health. Gandhi said: "You must chew your drinks and drink your foods."

All that I have said smacks of rigidity; this diet appears to be one of very stringent, restrictive discipline. Yet do not be seduced into fanaticism! And, above all, do not fall a victim to anxiety. Nothing is absolute save the laws of relativity and change. I cannot urge you enough to be flexible and unafraid; seek to know yourself and your needs.

The foods from yang to yin

△△△ = Very Yang
△△ = More Yang
△ = Yang

▽▽▽ = Very Yin
▽▽ = More Yin
▽ = Yin

ANIMAL AND FOWL

pheasant** △△△
egg* △△
turkey** △△
duck △△
partridge** △△

pigeon △
chicken** ▽
hare ▽▽
horse ▽▽

beef ▽▽
pork ▽▽
frog ▽▽
snail ▽▽

* Must be fertilized
** Must have been fed organic whole grain

FISH

caviar △△   sole △   carp ▽
red snapper △△   trout ▽   eel ▽
sardine △△   lobster ▽   octopus ▽
herring △△   halibut ▽   clam ▽
shrimp △△   mussel ▽   oyster ▽
salmon △

CEREALS

buckwheat △△   whole wheat △   barley ▽
millet △   rye ▽   corn ▽
rice △   oats ▽

VEGETABLES

burdock △△   endive △   bamboo shoots ▽▽
dandelion root △△   lettuce △   artichoke ▽▽
watercress △△   dandelion leaves △   spinach ▽▽
coltsfoot △△   cabbage (white) ▽   asparagus ▽▽
carrot △△   lentil ▽   cucumber ▽▽
pumpkin △△   beet ▽   beans (except
parsley △   celery ▽▽   azuki) ▽▽
onion △   cabbage (red) ▽▽   potato ▽▽▽
radish △   green peas ▽▽   sweet potato ▽▽▽
turnip △   garlic ▽▽   tomato ▽▽▽
kale △   mushroom ▽▽▽   eggplant ▽▽▽

DAIRY FOODS

goat cheese △△   Camembert ▽   cream cheese ▽▽▽
goat milk △△   milk ▽▽   sweet cream ▽▽▽
Dutch cheese △   margarine ▽▽▽   sour cream ▽▽▽
Roquefort △   butter ▽▽▽   yogurt ▽▽▽
Gruyere ▽

FRUITS

apple △△
strawberry △
chestnut △
cherry △
olive ▽
peach ▽▽
hazel nut ▽▽

cashew ▽▽
peanut ▽▽
almond ▽▽
pear ▽▽▽
melon ▽▽▽
orange ▽▽▽
fig ▽▽▽

banana ▽▽▽
grapefruit ▽▽▽
mango ▽▽▽
papaya ▽▽▽
pineapple ▽▽▽
lime ▽▽▽

MISCELLANEOUS

black sesame oil △
corn oil ▽
white sesame oil ▽
sunflower oil ▽

olive oil ▽▽
peanut oil ▽▽
safflower oil ▽▽
coconut oil ▽▽

margarine ▽▽▽
lard ▽▽▽
molasses ▽▽▽
honey ▽▽▽

BEVERAGES

ginseng △△△
mu tea △△
yannoh (Ohsawa coffee) △
kohkoh △
chicory △
bancha (common undyed Japanese tea) △

armoise (mugwort) △
menthol ▽
thyme ▽
water (deep well) ▽
soda ▽
mineral water ▽

beer ▽▽
wine ▽▽▽
champagne ▽▽▽
all sugared drinks ▽▽▽
fruit juice ▽▽▽
coffee ▽▽▽
tea (dyed) ▽▽▽

A quick summary of what you will learn

Here is a list of preferred foods and methods of cooking them:

GRAINS

Rice	In any form: boiled, fried, as cream, croquettes, dessert, etc.
Wheat	Bread, noodles, crepes, fritters, couscous, bulgur, chapati, cookies, pie crusts, cream soups and desserts, etc.
Barley	Cream, soup, bread, cookies, plain.
Oats	Cream, soup, cookies, pie crusts, desserts.
Millet	Is cooked very quickly. Cream, soup, boiled.

Buckwheat	Cream, fritters, boiled, cookies, bread when mixed with other cereals, croquettes, etc.
Rye	Cream, bread, cookies.

VEGETABLES (those we use the most)

Carrot	Sautéed, in soup, for pies, grated raw for salad, etc.
Onion	Sautéed, deep fried, in sauce, soup, pie, croquettes, etc.
Pumpkin	Sautéed, in soup, pies, desserts, baked, etc.
Cabbage	Sautéed, in soup.
Scallion	With fried rice, in croquettes, sautéed, in sauces, etc.
Turnip	Sautéed.
Watercress	Sautéed, in soup, in sandwiches, in salad, etc.
Burdock	Sautéed, in salad, in soup.
Endive	Sautéed, in salad.
Lettuce	Boiled, in salad, sautéed.
Parsley	Everywhere.

FISH

Sole	Broiled, boiled, sautéed with flour, deep fried.
Flounder	The same.
Swordfish	Broiled, deep fried.
Red snapper	Sautéed, cooked in pot with specific spices, barbecued with certain kinds of herbs.
Sardine	Sautéed, deep fried, not canned.

Shrimp	Sautéed with scallions and rice, deep fried, etc.
Salmon	Smoked, in sandwiches, baked, broiled.
Herring	In salt, very good in salad, broiled.

ANIMAL FOODS

All foods are permitted in this regime; a food is only forbidden by your body when it does not need it. Our senses are our guides; we must try to combine their signals with the needs of our body. It does not mean that we should not eat animal foods once in a while: when you meet your friends for the New Year, etc.

Preferred: Pheasant, eggs, turkey, duck, partridge, chicken, pigeon, lamb, sheep.

DAIRY PRODUCTS

A piece of goat cheese or roquefort (blue cheese) is very good in combination with an old wine. Why not?

FRUITS

Apples are the most recommendable, in any form: baked, sautéed, in pie, in sauce (homemade), etc.

Strawberries in pies and during the season; raw in salted water.

All fruits that grow around your town.

You can eat an orange in Morocco!

OILS

For cooking, the best are: sunflower, sesame, corn, olive.

For frying, you can use vegetable oil, which is more acid (yin).

Sesame oil is the best for pastry. Don't use it for deep frying; it is very fragile and spoils quickly.

SPICES

Some people may prefer not to use them. They do not wish to cover up the natural taste of vegetables.

Thyme	With millet, fish, as a drink (fresh, in leaf form).
Bay leaves	With fish, in soups.
Parsley	Raw, cooked, in soups, with fish, vegetables, with almost all foods.
Ginger	With fish, in cookies, soups. Very yin.
Nutmeg	Cookies, pies, vegetables, soups.
Coriander	Same use as nutmeg.
Lemon peel	For cookies, pies, crusts, desserts, drinks, etc.
Cinnamon	Desserts, cookies, drinks.
Vanilla	Desserts, like pies, custards, drinks.

DRINKS

Plants good for decoction:

Burdock root (dried)	Very yang. Good for rheumatism and ailments of the skin.
Gentian	Good for indigestion. Excellent for the stomach.
Mint	In case of acidity.
Anise	Good for airsickness.
Mugwort	Very efficient vermifuge. Accelerates menstruation.
Thyme	Stimulates digestion. Good for colds and asthma.

Sage	For indigestion. Very yang.
Rosemary	For the liver and circulation.

The daily drinks:

Mu tea	The most yang beverage. Can be used every day by yin people. Contains 16 plants.
Wheat tea	In summer; cold.
Dandelion coffee	Very yang. Good for yin people.
Ohsawa coffee	Very yang. Good stimulant.
Bancha tea	After your meals. For friends. Very delicious.

In the summer (once in a while):

Malt beer	Very yin. Very good for friends and happiness of an evening.
Muesli	Made with oatmeal, apples, raisins and lemon peels. Yin but very good. It is your whiskey.
Everything	In very small amounts; once in a great while. Avoid very cold drinks.

Remember, the most important thing is to chew. Quantity spoils quality. Your body operates astonishing changes. The ideal, according to George Ohsawa, is to eat only rice. But who is capable of eating only rice?

Eat a little bit of everything written about in this book and most of all enjoy it.

Before you dive into your pots

Relax!

Leave all unhappy thoughts at the door of your kitchen.

Always wash your hands before you start, like a surgeon.

Do not restrict yourself to exact timing. A fire might be stronger, a pot heavier. The liquid quantity might vary; a soup for 25 persons will take more time to cook than that for 4. There is a 15-minute difference in the boiling points of the two quantities.

Your judgment is important. The recipes we are giving will help to stir your imagination. Don't see them as fixed recipes.

Learn how to work alone and without help.

Cooking should not be a copy of a recipe but a creation in itself.

Do not leave your stove for too long. Stay near your work as much as possible.

A big secret: *sympathy*. Love what you do. If you are full of hatred, if you do not like anyone that day and like yourself even less, do not enter the kitchen; it is a sacred place where the man of tomorrow will be created. Don't forget that only high monks in the East were allowed to enter or work in the kitchen!

The golden rule is that the pleasure to create makes things more succulent. Don't load yourself with a giant utensil to stir or serve food. One gesture, a particular attention to any preparation, is like the wind in the field which sweetly blows and gives to the ear of corn its beauty.

Appetite is often influenced by a good presentation of food. Therefore use contrast. Grains are good friends with colors. One agrees with green; another prefers red. For example, the green of parsley makes a bowl of rice happier. A radish refreshes and vivifies the whiteness of millet; a fresh leaf of lettuce does wonders for the brown of fried fish. An alive color on a brown cereal is like a song in your heart.

Every dish should contain its yin and yang, not only chemically, but in the presentation and consistency of the components. Rice, buckwheat and noodles in the same plate are not too exciting to the appetite. Croquettes, fritters, crusty ends in the soup, crusty pies make for diversion.

All depends first on your actual condition. A Number 7 regime, which means only cereals, is not as rich as the 4th and 5th regimes (in Introduction).

Rice and buckwheat can be mixed or presented together in different ways.

Millet and buckwheat do not agree at all. They are both too yang and have individual tastes that do not blend. But as buckwheat rebuffs miso, millet welcomes it.

Rice and azuki: very good.

Millet and azuki: very good.

Watercress and rice and dandelion and rice are examples of good marriages.

Any wheat agrees with onion. Couscous happily accepts this sweet vegetable. The same applies to turnips.

Good associations: Carrot-onion, cabbage-onion, zucchini-onion, zucchini-pepper (very yin), etc.

There are a thousand and one ways to accommodate the cereals which you do not now like. Be patient and you will appreciate them all.

And now to your pots.

Grains—cereals

Rice, the king of kings

Brown rice has seven skins. The outside skin is very resistant to chemical effects but is weak physically; it should be husked carefully. The quality of the grain changes as soon as the skin is broken.

The rice you usually find in the market is not satisfactory to your needs. Many debilitating operations are involved before it becomes white. Processors rub it, polish it, sometimes stain it and end by covering it with talc and glucose.

Brown rice contains 9.17% protein; white rice contains only 8.85%.

Brown rice contains 2.40% fat; white rice, 0.60%.

In white rice silicium, magnesium, phosphorous lose 30% to 50% of their original values. The antineuritic vitamin B1 disappears. The same thing happens to calcium and other minerals.

Brown rice is the food that comes closest to the ratio 5 parts of potassium to 1 of sodium. All foods having proportions of potassium greater than 5 are more yin; those under 5, more yang. The ratio of potassium to sodium in a potato is 512 to 1; in a banana, 850 to 1.

RICE

Use 1 cup brown rice (washed) for 2 cups cold water and 1/2 teaspoon sea salt. Allow ingredients to come to a rapid boil and then cook slowly over a low flame in a covered pot for 45 minutes or more. Ideally, one should cook this cereal until the bottom of the pot is slightly scorched. The yellow part is most yang, the best, because it is richest in minerals.

When rice is cooked in a pressure cooker, use 1 to 1-1/2 parts of water to 1 part of rice. After boiling, use a very low flame for 20 to 25 minutes. Turn off heat and let stand. Remove cover after 10 to 20 minutes.

SAKURA RICE

Before putting washed brown rice on to boil, add 1 tablespoonful tamari to the water. The amount of tamari that suits your taste is an individual matter—start with 1 tablespoonful per cup of rice.

ADUKI RICE

Tiny red delicious aduki beans require longer cooking than does rice so it is well to bring the beans to a boil in a separate pot before putting the rice on. Again, proportion is an individual matter. Start with 1 part beans to 8 parts rice. Add the partly cooked beans to the rice and salted water and boil in the usual way. Rice and beans is a principal food in many parts of the world. It survives as a soulfood staple in the repertoire of the best Negro cooks in the United States.

GOMUKU RICE

Prepare a small amount of onion, carrot, leek, parsley, garlic the way the Japanese call "nituke," which is detailed in another section of the book. Try to time your cooking so the vegetables are done about the same time as the boiled rice is ready. Mix them together before serving.

FRIED RICE WITH SCALLIONS

The best way to prepare fried rice is in a Chinese frying pan or wok. Cut 5 or 6 scallions into small pieces and sauté them either in corn oil or in sesame oil. Do not take more than a minute or two to sauté them, otherwise the scallions will lose their bright green color and decompose. Add boiled rice immediately, breaking any lumps with a wooden spoon, and mixing the rice well with the scallions. All this takes only a few minutes over a medium flame. Add a mixture of 1/2 water and 1/2 tamari—quantity to your taste. Stir again and serve hot.

FRIED RICE FOR GUESTS

>   2 carrots, cut into tiny cubes
>   4 scallions, finely chopped
>   1 onion, medium size, minced
>   6 shrimp, large, cut into small pieces
>   3 cabbage leaves, shredded
>   4 cups boiled rice
>   tamari

Use preferably a Chinese frying pan. First, sauté the onion over a high flame, turning constantly until golden in color. Add scallions and right after that, add the cabbage, mixing and turning until it is quite limp. Then mix in the pieces of shrimp Carrots take a longer time to soften than the other vegetables. Cook the carrots separately for 10 minutes and add them to the rest of the vegetables.

(Don't be frightened by the need to cook things separately; you will be amazed to discover how helpful it is. In fact, it often gives better results, and truly it does not take more time.) Now add the boiled rice, breaking up any lumps with a wooden spoon, and a mixture of tamari and water. Keep turning and mixing for a few minutes. Serve immediately.

BROWN RICE CROQUETTES

Mix nituke vegetables or nituke scallions with boiled rice, add a little salt and enough whole wheat flour and water so the croquettes hold together. They may be pan fried or deep fried in oil. For special occasions, the croquettes can be dipped in beaten egg and then rolled in rice cream powder (recipe given a little later), more whole wheat flour, or even cornmeal. This is a quick way of serving what all cookbooks call "leftovers."

SESAME RICE

Toast a couple of tablespoonfuls of whole sesame seeds for a few minutes on the top of the stove until they turn brown. Then add them to washed brown rice and water before boiling as usual. The proportion will depend on your taste. Usually 1 tablespoon is enough for 1 cup rice.

CHESTNUT RICE

Boil or roast a few chestnuts until they are tender. If you cut a slit in the rounded side of the chestnut, the way French street vendors do, they will roast quickly and the outer and inner shells will come off as easy as a peanut shell. Take the tender chestnuts—in proportions of about 1 to 5 in relation to the rice—add them to the rice, salt and water and boil the rice mixture as usual. The chestnuts blend with the brown rice in a delectable combination of flavors.

COUSCOUS RICE

Chick peas, pois chiche, garbanzo beans, Egyptian beans—whatever you call them—are a perfect addition to rice. Handle them in the same way as chestnuts or aduki beans.

The chick peas should be soaked overnight in warm water, boiled a little in advance of the rice, then added to the rice and water to finish cooking jointly.

Or, completely cooked chick peas, sautéed with a little onion, can be mixed with rice already cooked.

RICE BALLS

This is another way of using cooked rice to advantage. Prepare a solution of cold salted water, about 1 teaspoonful salt to 1 cup of water. Dip your hands in the solution to avoid making a sticky mess of handling the rice. Take about 2 heaping teaspoons cooked rice and press into shape like ping-pong balls. Then the fun begins.

- Roll the balls in roasted sesame seeds.
- Roll the balls in mashed cooked aduki beans.
- Toast sheets of nori, a seaweed we will discuss later, over the open flame until they change color, and wrap the seaweed around the balls.
- Take a sliver of dried umeboshi plum and put it in the center of the rice ball. This not only enhances the flavor, but serves as a natural preservative. The rice balls will not spoil for days even in summer, and make perfect portable snacks.
- Mix the rice with nituke vegetables or aduki beans.
- Drop the rice balls into hot oil and fry them.

RICE CREAM

>   4 tablespoons rice cream
>   3 cups water, cold
>   3/4 teaspoon salt

Infinity Food Co. makes a fine rice cream; it is already toasted. Put the rice cream into a cold saucepan. Add just 1 cup of the water and the salt. Place pan over a high flame; stir mixture until smooth. When thick, add another cup of water. Repeat until all the water has been added. Lower the flame and simmer for 20 minutes. If cream becomes too thick, add more water and increase salt by 1/4 teaspoon per cup of water added. Rice cream is a breakfast cereal. If serving to children, simmer 1 hour or longer over a controlled flame—i.e., with a flame diffuser or asbestos sheet over the flame.

You can use buckwheat flour, barley flour, kokkoh, millet flour, etc. in the same way.

RICE PIE

Prepare a batch of pie crust according to the recipe given later in this book. Fill the unbaked pie shell with cooked rice, to which you add nituke vegetables in the proportion of 5 to 1. Add a little water and a dash of tamari. Cover the pie with a top crust and bake for 1/2 hour or so in a 350° oven until the crust is golden.

These are merely a few of the directions one can go in fancying up plain brown rice. The possibilities are unlimited, depending on the season and the availability of complementary foods. Once you have your kitchen stocked with macrobiotic staples, and begin to react instinctively to other foods as they fit into the scale of yin and yang, you improvise and improve.

Try with watercress, dandelion, chick peas and carrots, alone or in combinations.

KASHA WITH VEGETABLE GRAVY

2 cups buckwheat groats
1 cup onions, minced
1 cup cabbage, shredded
1/2 cup carrots, diced
1/2 cup whole wheat flour, sifted
7 cups water
2 tablespoons tamari
1 tablespoon tahini
2 tablespoons sesame oil

Sauté the groats in 1 tablespoon oil, stirring constantly, until they are browned and nutty. Cool bottom of pan, add 5 cups water and salt and bring to a boil. Lower flame, cover and simmer for just 5 minutes; turn off flame. In a skillet, heat 1 tablespoon oil. Sauté in it the onions, cabbage, and carrots. In a deep saucepan, dry-toast the whole wheat flour lightly, stirring constantly. Cool bottom of pan and add 2 cups water. Bring to a boil and then add the tamari, tahini and sautéed vegetables, stirring constantly. When mixture begins to thicken, turn down flame, cook for just 15 minutes and turn off flame. Prepare casserole dish by greasing lightly with sesame oil and heating. Pour vegetable gravy over kasha and bake at 300° for 1/2 hour.

BUCKWHEAT CROQUETTES

1 cup buckwheat groats
4 cups boiling water
1 tablespoon sea salt
1 cup whole wheat flour
2 tablespoons sesame oil
2 small, grated onions
4 or 5 scallions, minced
1 handful parsley, chopped
1 egg, optional

In a deep saucepan, dry-toast buckwheat groats till brown and nutty. Add boiling water and salt and cook 20 minutes. Let cool and add the whole wheat flour. Heat oil in a skillet and sauté onions, lightly. Allow onions to cool. Add cooled onions and minced scallions to kasha and flour. If an egg is used, beat and add. Knead ingredients to firm consistency. Form croquettes to desired shape and size, and dip into whole wheat flour or oat flakes. Fry in pan, using just enough oil to cover the bottom of the pan. When browned, remove croquettes and place on white paper towel to absorb oil.

KASHA VARNITCHKES

>2 cups buckwheat groats
>8 cups boiling water
>2 teaspoons sea salt
>2 tablespoons sesame oil
>4 onions, minced
>1/2 pound whole wheat noodles

Dry-toast buckwheat groats until brown and nutty. Add water and salt and cook 20 minutes. In a deep saucepan, heat oil and sauté onions till golden; mix with cooked kasha. Boil noodles, drain and let stand for a few minutes. Mix with kasha and simmer together 5 minutes.

FRIED KASHA

Cook buckwheat groats. Chop up 2 or 3 scallions and sauté them in heated oil for 1 or 2 minutes. Add cooked kasha, turn and stir for 5 minutes over medium flame. Do not forget the salt.

KASHA NOODLES GRATINEE

In individual Pyrex dishes put a layer of cooked kasha, then a layer of noodles. Over them pour sauce bechamel (*see* Sauces) generously. Put under broiler for 10 to 15 minutes.

Serve with chopped parsley. Instead of sauce bechamel, you can use grated swiss cheese. Don't forget it's animal food, but once in a while it's good.

Couscous

In Morocco where I was raised, the national dish was couscous, a hand-processed type of wheat cereal. It is prepared differently in Tunisia, Algeria and Morocco and there are several schools of thought on the best way of cooking it.

It is customary for invited guests to gather around a "kessria," which is a huge clay pot, and serve themselves without utensils other than their bare hands. The divers form small balls of the couscous and pop them into their mouths as fast as they can. An important concomitant of this procedure is a loud and healthy belch, which is considered a necessary social obligation due the host for his largess. With the advancing civilization, metal utensils are supplanting the natural ones, and the usual table silver is common.

The traditional hand-processing of couscous entails long and complicated preparation. I will show you how to simplify and shorten this preparation after first describing the old way.

It is essential to buy the best available brand of couscous (obviously of Moroccan origin since I come from there!). However, if that is unavailable, the Tunisian variety is acceptable. A pound (preferably boxed) is sufficient for 4 people. A special couscous double pot is necessary for good results. The perforated upper pot, in which the couscous is placed, receives steam from the lower one; this indirect steaming produces a very special flavor.

Soak 1-1/2 cups chick peas overnight in lukewarm water. Drain and reserve liquid. Boil 2 quarts water in a pan. Allow it to cook for about an hour over a low flame. Meanwhile, pour **couscous** from the box into a large deep platter. Pour 1 cup water over it and fluff it for a few minutes with your fingers in an upward movement. Allow it to stand for about 10 minutes so that the couscous absorbs the water. Then roll the grains between the palms of both hands, until the grains are separated from each other. Pour the water in which the chick peas were soaked into the lower pot. Put the couscous into the upper pot, place it on the lower pot and cook over a medium flame for 45 minutes. The steam from the lower pot will penetrate the upper one containing the couscous.

Slice 4 carrots, 4 onions, 1 leek and 1 pound pumpkin into fairly large pieces. Add to the boiling water in the lower pot at the same time as the chick peas. Add sufficient salt for taste.

When the steam has heated the couscous, remove it to a large receptacle and let stand 10 to 15 minutes. Once again roll the couscous between your palms (if you can stand the heat); otherwise, bruise with a wooden spoon. Add 1 cup lukewarm water and keep stirring while you add 2 tablespoons olive oil and a little bit of salt. Return the couscous to the upper pot and resteam it for an additional 20 minutes. It is ready after that! It can remain on a low flame for a few hours.

Serve it this way: place the couscous affectionately on the serving platter and then place the vegetables over it. Scoop liquid from the lower pot and pour over the platter.

ANOTHER WAY TO PREPARE COUSCOUS

Place dry couscous in a strainer and pour boiling water over it, then drain and put into a large and deep platter. Taste it to determine the consistency and flavor. If the couscous is hard and dry, add 1/2 cup or more boiling water. Roll couscous quickly between your palms. Add salt and 2 tablespoons olive oil, and place the couscous in the upper pot of the cooker. Vegetables must, of course, be cooked as previously indicated.

STILL ANOTHER WAY OF PREPARING COUSCOUS

Pour 1 pound couscous into a pressure cooker with an equal volume of water. Add salt. Cook over high flame for 3 minutes, then reduce simmer for an additional 5 minutes. Don't remove the lid from the pressure cooker for at least 8 minutes. Prepare vegetables as previously explained or, if you wish, they may be sautéed first, adding a little water later.

FRIED COUSCOUS

If you have some couscous left over, you can make a delicious dish by merely sautéing it. Sauté a handful of scallions (finely chopped) for about 2 minutes. Add a sufficient amount of couscous for one or two persons and stir for 5 minutes.

It's so good! I discovered this purely by accident.

Crêpes and pancakes

The pancake has made a big comeback recently in the United States where drive-in pancake parlors specialize in perversions of the classic frontier dish, dressing it up with milk, butter, jam, fruit syrup, ice cream and all the accoutrements of a banana split.

In France, tradition has kept the crêpes sold on the streets of Paris much closer to the classic dish that was a holy day treat in the Middle Ages. The crêpe is associated with two religious holidays: Chandeleur or Candlemas Day, Feb. 2, which is the feast of the purification of the Virgin, and Mardi Gras, the carnival day before the beginning of Lent.

After French peasants parade in the streets, candles in hand, singing hymns, they return to their firesides where, after a day of fasting, they have crêpes made of rye flour, salt, water and eggs. Once this was the only dessert within reach of the man in the street. The flipping of the crêpes in the skillet was a skill of great virtuosity and superstition, even as the flipping of a coin appeals to the gambling instinct.

The classic French batter recipe hasn't changed in centuries. Neither have the secrets for making successful crêpes.

There are 7 important factors in the making of a successful crêpe:

>the batter
>the time it takes to make the batter
>the quality of the pan
>the quantity of oil on the pan
>the fire
>the time it takes to cook the crêpe
>and how to turn the crêpe

The batter can be made with whole wheat flour, unbleached flour or buckwheat flour.

BASIC BATTER

Use 3 volumes of water for 1 volume of flour. Add salt to taste. Mix and let it stand for at least 2 hours. The pan must be cast iron, smooth and even. The pan edge must be low.

Heat the pan well. Oil it with a brush or with a piece of cloth. Before adding the batter, lower the flame to 1/3 of its possible height. The quantity of the batter changes according to the dimension of the pan. For a 9-inch pan (diameter of the bottom), use 7 ounces of batter.

As you pour in the batter with your left hand, keep turning the pan clockwise to spread evenly the batter over the pan.

Time: 7 to 10 minutes for the first side; 3 to 5 minutes for the second. Exact timing depends on the thickness of the crêpe.

Before turning the crêpe over, try to detach it with a very flat spatula.

CRÊPE DE SARASIN
(Buckwheat crêpe)

The proportion of water to flour is 3 to 1. The flour must be very fine. Add salt, 1 beaten egg and mix. Let the batter stand for at least 2 hours. Heat the pan and oil it. Pour the batter into the pan, and keep turning the pan clockwise until the batter is spread evenly.

STUFFINGS

You can stuff a crêpe with various things. A crêpe may serve as an hors d'oeuvre or as a dessert if it is filled with a preparation which agrees with its consistency. A dry, hard filling would not be appropriate. By looking at the crêpe, one understands that only a soft and delicate filling is welcome. Here are the best ingredients you can use for an hors d'oeuvre: sautéed carrots, carrots and onions, scallions, endive, zucchini, zucchini and onions, onions, dandelion, watercress, etc.

As a dessert, stuff the crêpe with a sliced baked apple or an apple sautéed in oil with raisins and toasted almonds, applesauce, etc.

Millet

MILLET VEGETABLE STEW

1 tablespoon sesame oil
1/2 cup onion, sliced
1/2 cup carrot, sliced
1/2 cup pumpkin, sliced
1 cup millet
3 cups water
2 teaspoons tamari

Toast hulled millet (millet with the hull takes interminable cooking). In a pressure cooker, first sauté in oil the onion, then the carrot and pumpkin. Cool the pan and add the millet, water and tamari. Pressure-cook for 20 minutes, using a very low flame but making sure top jiggles throughout cooking. Do not put pressure cooker under cold water to bring down the pressure; let it drop slowly.

GRATIN DE MILLET

This requires the same preparation as the preceding recipe, but use 4 cups of water instead of 3. Cook the millet, then put it in baking dish 1 inch deep, pouring bechamel sauce over the millet. Bake in a 350° oven or under broiler for 20 minutes.

STUFFED ONION WITH MILLET

Scoop out large onions from the top and put them into salted boiling water for 5 or 10 minutes. Remove onions, drain, and stuff with cooked millet and vegetables. For more flavor, add a pinch of nutmeg, a few bread crumbs and tahini. Bake in 350° oven 15 minutes or more.

Breads

YEASTED BREAD

Chewable, yeast is yin. Yeasted bread is usually baked for parties and gatherings. I personally attended only three or four parties the last year!

> 2 cups whole wheat flour
> 2 cups rye flour
> 2 tablespoons corn oil
> 1/2 teaspoon salt
> 1/2 teaspoon self-rising yeast, dissolved
>   in 1/4 cup hot water

Mix flours with oil and salt in a large bowl. Work with your hands until the oil is evenly distributed and not lumpy. Let stand 1/2 hour. Mix in the yeast with your hands. Add water until the dough rolls off the sides of the bowl. Flour the dough and put into an oiled bread pan. Let sit at least 1 hour. For better results, let sit overnight. Bake in oven at 375°, approximately 1 to 1-1/2 hours.

VARIATIONS

1) Whole wheat flour
   Unbleached white flour
   Corn or soy flour (in small quantity, yin)

2) Buckwheat flour
   Soy flour (small quantity)
   Unbleached white flour

3) Whole wheat flour
   Unbleached white flour

4) Rye flour
   Unbleached white flour

UNYEASTED BREAD

Barely chewable! By the way, have you visited your dentist lately? You need good teeth to enjoy this miraculous bread—the more you chew it, the better it is.

2 cups whole wheat flour
1 cup buckwheat flour
1 cup cornmeal
1/2 cup soy flour
1 teaspoon salt
2 tablespoons oil
1 tablespoon sesame butter

Mix flours, salt and oil together in a bowl. Work very well with your hands until oil is evenly distributed. Let stand 1 hour. (If you want your bread to rise, let it stand over night.) Add water and work very well with your hands until dough is sticky and almost elastic. Form into loaf, flour and place in an oiled pan. Let stand 1/2 hour. Bake in oven at approximately 375° for 1 to 1-1/2 hours.

VARIATIONS

       1) 4 cups whole wheat flour
          2 cups buckwheat flour
          2 cups cornmeal
          2 cups cooked rice
          1-1/2 teaspoon salt
          10 tablespoons oil
          1/4 cup roasted sesame seeds

Bake as above, sprinkling sesame seeds on top.

       2) 2 cups whole wheat flour
          1/2 cup buckwheat groats
          1 tablespoon oil
          1/2 teaspoon salt

3) Any cooked grain such as rice, buckwheat or millet may be added to the bread dough. Have fun—use your own judgment in mixing other flours together.

BREADSTICKS

>2 cups whole wheat flour
>2 cups unbleached flour
>2 tablespoons oil
>1 teaspoon salt
>2 to 3 cups water

Mix flours as for bread. Dough should be fairly firm. Let sit 1 hour and roll on floured board as for pie crust, 1/4 inch thick and 6 inches long. Roll sticks in sesame seeds and bake in oven at 375°, approximately 20 minutes, until outside is turning brown.

CHAPATI

Chapati is a quickly made delicious bread, perfect for traveling and picnics.

Mix equal portions of whole wheat flour and corn flour. Salt to taste. Add water until dough rolls off the sides of the bowl and is not sticking to your fingers. Flatten dough in your hands and place in an oiled pan. Cook 10 minutes for each side over a medium flame.

Also try buckwheat and unbleached white flour. Make the chapati very thin.

The children of grain

"Master!" called another disciple, "is there any difference between a child who eats grain and a child who eats animal food?"

The master lit a cigarette.

"Aha! Is there any difference?" The Master was silent for a long moment. Those who were at his feet that day were accustomed to his silences. They waited, anticipating either facetiousness or simple, straightforward wisdom.

"The difference is very great. A child who eats grains and vegetables has a better memory and better understanding than the child who eats mainly meat. His mind is clearer, more agile. His answers in school are more precise. His decisions, in anything he undertakes, are very quick. I would be very curious to know the IQ of the one and the other.

"No child should be fed with exactly the same foods as its parents. The child, for instance, needs less salt and more water than an adult. Parents are the sculptors of their child until its adolescence; after adolescence, the boy is his own artist."

Secondary foods

Nituke

In the macrobiotic cooking scheme, vegetables are a secondary food, intended to be served in small amounts, mainly as a seasoning or garnish for your principal food. But good things come in small packages; two tablespoons of vegetables cooked in the Japanese fashion can be the jewel of the meal. Nituke and tempura, the basic Japanese methods of preparing vegetables, are designed to make each morsel of each vegetable important. Properly prepared, there is more flavor in a small sliver of nituke carrot than there is in a whole mess of frozen, thawed, stewed, brewed and tattooed vegetables out of a can or the corner supermarket deep-freeze.

The nituke method of cooking vegetables has lately come into fashion as a promotion of the vegetable oil manufacturers and the margarine makers. But what they leave out is that nituke always starts with fresh vegetables, organically grown if possible and used only in season. You will learn in your shopping to pass by the gorgeously manicured, chemically treated, highly colored vegetables. Just as you learn to yearn for an apple with a worm in it—the natural trademark of fruit free of chemicals and insecticides—so you will learn to spring to attention and direct all your impulse shopping to the tired, forlorn, limp vegetables on the way to the refuse bin. Vegetable fatigue merely means that some of the water has evaporated. In most cases the flavor is improved, not impaired. It will take less cooking to prepare them properly. Never peel any vegetable. Give it a good scrubbing, that's all. No soaking in water to "freshen them up."

For nituke vegetables, it is best to learn to wield a heavy Japanese knife. With this and a wooden block, you can slice them up in properly tiny morsels. For nituke, first slice root vegetables diagonally very thin; then slice the diagonal pieces into matchstick pieces. Use a tiny amount of vegetable oil: corn, olive, sunflower or sesame oil. Until you get used to it, sesame oil is best used in small quantities to spike the other oils. (For deep frying tempura, where larger quantities of oil are necessary and economy is a factor, you may use corn oil and sesame oil combined. But any economy in this area is what is known in Yiddish as "kishka gelt" or stomach money, a poor place for any but the most unavoidable economies.)

After you sauté the vegetables in the oil, add a tiny amount of water, just enough to avoid burning, then a little sea salt. Cover the vegetables and cook over a low flame until they are wilted, until all the moisture and liquid have evaporated. At the end add soya sauce to taste.

All nituke properly prepared is a little salty, so get used to it. Practically any vegetable can be prepared in this way, from yams, the most yang, to mushrooms which are about as yin as you can comfortably experiment. Many of the root vegetables work fine in combinations. Onion and garlic are the most sociable of vegetables, mixing with anything to advantage, as everybody knows.

Pearl Buck, after years in the Orient, once said it might be worth more than all the gold in Fort Knox if American women could learn to cook vegetables Oriental fashion "without water and waste."

In fact, there are two ways to make a nituke. The first consists of cutting the vegetables in small strips and cooking them by staying near the fire all the time during the operation. It is the fastest way. The second way takes longer. This time, the vegetables are larger in size; you can put them in to cook and leave the kitchen if you wish.

1st METHOD

Delicately cut your vegetables in thin strips (almost like matches). Heat 1 tablespoon of oil in a frying pan, put the vegetables in the pan and stir constantly. Cook 5 to 10 minutes over high flame. Reduce to a medium flame and cook 10 to 15 minutes longer. Stir constantly. A few minutes before the end, add soy sauce and a tiny bit of water.

2nd METHOD

Cut your vegetables into 1 x 1/2-inch pieces. Heat 1 tablespoon oil in a frying pan. Add the vegetables and stir 5 minutes over a high flame. Add 1 cup water, and salt. Reduce the flame. Cover the pot or pan. Cook 30 to 40 minutes over low flame. If the water evaporates, add a few drops; don't over-moisten.

CARROT SESAME

Carrot nituke becomes something else again when dusted with roasted sesame seeds. Add 1 teaspoonful sesame seeds for 2 average-size carrots after you have added the tamari soya sauce. More or less seeds may be used, depending on your taste. Then cook for another few minutes, stirring well.

DANDELION NITUKE

Dandelion blossoms can be used to make a delicious white wine. The leaves are used by some gourmets in salads. And Greeks always have them available as a hot or cold vegetable. For most people, however, the beautiful dandelion is a suburban curse, second to crabgrass as a menace to the unending green of well manicured lawns.

Be cautious about picking dandelions in some neighborhoods. They may be more full of chemicals than some of the vegetables in the market. Pick dandelion leaves from your own lawn or some rustic spot. Pull up the whole plant—roots and all. The roots are delicious cooked separately. Wash the leaves well, cut them into small pieces and make a nituke, adding salt and tamari soy sauce.

To cooking dandelion roots, wash them well, but do not peel. Cut into thin round pieces. Cook well in oil, using about 1 tablespoon oil to 1 cup chopped dandelion root. When the dandelion roots are nearly done, add 1/2 teaspoon of salt and a dash of tamari.

Dandelion root nituke is especially recommended for sufferers from arthritis, rheumatism, cardiac diseases.

ENDIVE

Most endive is still imported from Belgium, which makes it out of bounds in the United States. Try to find the native variety organically grown (some health food shops sometimes have it); it is delicious served nituke-style.

It is sufficient to cut each endive in half lengthwise. Cook quite quickly in oil. Add salt and tamari, and serve.

BROCCOLI

Slice a stalk of broccoli into small pieces, sauté in oil, add a little water and cook nituke-style, adding salt and tamari just before serving.

CELERY

Celery, being relatively yin and more potent when cooked than raw, lends itself to combinations with other vegetables, especially scallions.

BURDOCK

Burdock is more difficult to find, and takes longer to cook than almost any other vegetable. Because of its fantastic medicinal properties, it is usually available in most macrobiotic shops and health food stores. It is a long, almost black, root, longer and skinnier than the salsify. A good bit of muscle power is needed to scrub burdock adequately. Because burdock is very tough to cut, the best way is to shave it as one would sharpen a pencil. Burdock keeps for long periods without refrigeration.

Because its taste is at first a little strange, it is best to introduce burdock in combination with a more familiar vegetable.

Sauté the shavings in a little vegetable oil and keep cooking until the pieces change color slightly. Then add carrots and continue as if you were preparing carrot nituke, cooking with a tiny amount of water. Add salt and tamari just before removing from fire.

ONIONS

Onions are great in combination with carrots, cabbage or almost any vegetable. They are also very tasteful cooked alone. Prepared as nituke, they have a completely different taste; the addition of salt and tamari makes them sweeter. The secret in preparing a delicious onion nituke is to cook the vegetable over a very low flame.

PARSNIPS

Parsnips can be handled exactly like carrots, in combination with onion or with roasted sesame seeds.

TURNIPS

This principal food of "Tobacco Road" comes out as sweet as can be when handled nituke-fashion, sautéed in oil or combined with onion. Salt and tamari are added just before cooking is complete.

WATERCRESS

One of the most yang of vegetables, relegated largely to salads or decorative garnishes in the United States, watercress is infinitely superior to the vaunted spinach among green vegetables.

Chop the stalks and leaves into fine pieces and sauté in oil. Like celery, watercress has a very high water content, so no additional water need be added when cooked carefully. Salt to taste or use tamari only.

STRING BEANS

String beans are relatively yin, so it is best to forget about them —if you are too yin—until your health is well established. Then for a once-in-a-while treat, cook them whole in a small amount of oil, removing only the tips. After the beans have wilted and shriveled, add tamari, a bit more than usual to yang-ize them some more. A pinch of garlic powder gives a delicious taste. You can add it at the beginning just before putting the string beans in the pan.

THREE VEGETABLES NITUKE

Soak chick peas overnight. Drain and boil gently in fresh water for 30 minutes. Salt to taste. When cooked, the skins should not split; if they do, you will have a puree after the next operation:

Cut carrots and onions into tiny pieces and sauté them together. Drain the cooked chick peas, and add them to the cooking nituke. Add salt to taste and cook over a low flame 20 minutes.

LEAF VEGETABLES

Lettuce, kale and cabbage can also be prepared as nituke. If you like garlic (yin), a sliver or two of finely chopped garlic may be added to almost any nituke.

Seaweed

HIZIKI

The first time I ate seaweed, at a friend's home in Paris, I closed my eyes and said to myself: "These people are kidding me, it's a joke!" When later I was told that it wasn't a joke, I thought the host was somewhat out of his mind. But now I recommend hiziki!

Try it; it is good for you. As for the taste—you'll get used to it, and eventually even love it.

> 4 ounces Hiziki
> Water to cover
> 2 tablespoons sesame oil
> 10 tablespoons soy sauce for cooking
> tamari to taste when served

Hiziki is the only seaweed served exclusively as a vegetable. To prepare, rinse in cold water, changing water twice. Then, allow to soak for about 15 minutes. Do not discard the soaking water; use it for cooking. Cut hiziki into 2-inch lengths. Heat the oil in a deep saucepan, and sauté the hiziki. Cool the bottom of the pan and add the water used for soaking. Bring to a rapid boil and add the tamari. Turn down the flame and simmer without a cover for about 1 hour until most of the liquid is evaporated.

HIZIKI WITH LOTUS or CARROTS

The best way to prepare hiziki is with lotus root (when in season). Dried lotus may also be used as well as carrots or sesame seeds. If you use lotus, use the same amount as hiziki. If you use carrots, use a little less than the amount of hiziki. One tablespoon toasted sesame seeds may be used to 4 ounces hiziki (recipe above), adding after the hiziki and water reach a boil. Prepare the lotus or carrot by first scrubbing with a vegetable brush; do not remove the skin but cut out any decayed part. Cut lengthwise into thin, 2-inch long strips. If you use dried lotus, first soak overnight; discard water. Sauté lotus or carrot in oil and then add hiziki. The rest of the recipe is the same as in cooking plain hiziki above.

WAKAME

Wakame is used in the following ways:

1) In miso soup (recipe in Soup section).
2) It can be deep fried or toasted over flame until crispy, and eaten as a condiment.
3) After soaking in water for 10 minutes, chop and cook with tamari and salt, using a little water.
4) Soak in water 10 minutes, chop and cook with miso paste, using a little water. Scallions may be added.
5) A summer preparation: after the wakame is soaked and chopped, cook in a very small amount of lemon juice with a bit of water.

NORI

The only preparation required for nori is toasting. Hold a nori sheet about 4 to 6 inches above a flame and wave gently until it starts to "crinkle." The principal use for nori is in making rice balls. Toasted nori can also be crumbled and used as a garnish.

Tempura

Such a smog of mystique has been stirred up around the subject of tempura that even experienced cooks have been known to panic when faced with the hot oil and the cool batter, or else to duck the challenge completely.

Some gourmets who bar-fly around the tempura bars in fancy Japanese restaurants will tell you that the secrets of tempura are handed down from Japanese cooks to Japanese cooks and they cannot be bribed into parting with them.

Never mind. Tempura is simple. Trial and error will eventually make anyone a master of the art. Even if your tempura is less than perfect, it is almost always edible. It is out of these interesting failures that you will learn your own tricks.

Tempura is a very simple process. Vegetables and/or shellfish are dipped in batter, or mixed with batter and deep fried in vegetable oil—corn, sesame, or sunflower oil, or a mixture of any vegetable oils spiked with a little sesame oil. A quart of oil is a convenient amount to work with. It can be filtered and saved for several batches. If it becomes crumb-y and cloudy, it can always be cleared at the end of a frying by tossing in an umeboshi plum, which acts as a precipitant.

For frying, use about 3 inches of oil in the deep fryer and heated to 350° or a little higher.

The batter is just as simple. There is no one perfect batter for tempura. There are many combinations, depending on the kind of flour used. Usually the best proportion is 1 cup of flour to 1-1/4 cups of cold water. But even this is not rigid. Sometimes, for beginners, it is easier to work with a slightly thicker batter. But the batter must be cool—use ice-cold water—and the oil should be hot.

The vegetables or shellfish should also be cooled; otherwise the batter quickly warms up from contact. Some people work with an ice cube in their batter.

For best results, some experts insist the batter should be mixed just before using. Others swear the results are better if the batter stands for 15 minutes. Try it both ways, take your choice.

If you are working with a very yang vegetable or shellfish, use whole wheat flour mixed with unbleached flour. If you are working with vegetables or shellfish which are more yin, increase the proportion of whole wheat flour or make the batter with only buckwheat flour, which is more yang.

It is difficult at first to judge how much tempura batter is needed to fry the amount of vegetables or shellfish you intend to use. You will be surprised how much batter you use. This is one of the most subtle facets of tempura: it increases the ratio of cereals to vegetables amazingly. Before you know it, a cup of flour has been used to prepare just a few vegetables. By cutting the vegetables fine, you increase the surfaces to which your batter will adhere.

BASIC BATTER

You can vary this basic batter by mixing buckwheat with white unbleached flour, rye and whole wheat flour or buckwheat flour with rice flour. You can trim the amount of water a little and use a well beaten fertilized egg.

    1 cup whole wheat flour
    1 to 1-1/4 cups cold water
    1/2 teaspoon sea salt
    1 egg, optional

Drop shellfish such as shrimp, mussels or oysters that are slippery to handle, into a sack with a few tablespoons of flour, and shake them until they are dusted. This thin coating will make them easier to handle and cause the batter to adhere and cover completely. This also works with vegetables that have been salted in advance and are slippery from loss of water.

If you run out of vegetables or shellfish and have batter left, drop it by the spoonful into the hot oil and fry it. It is like a miniature popover, delicious.

Instead of cold water, for frying oysters, try making a tempura batter out of the liquid from the oysters. For frying shrimp, use a stock made by boiling the shells of the shrimp for 15 minutes in water salted to taste. For mussels, use the stock made from steaming the mussels.

There is literally nothing that does not submit beautifully to this mode of cooking. To prove it, start with a throw-away vegetable such as the tops of carrots. Yes, carrot tops. Or watercress. Or take tempura from A to Z, apples to zucchini. (Apples are covered in many recipes in the Dessert section.)

CARROT TOPS

Group the tops of carrots into a miniature bouquet, dust them with salt, dip in batter and drop them into the deep oil.

CARROT ROOTS

Cut the carrots very thin, about 1 inch long and the thickness of kitchen matchsticks. Salt and cool them. Mix a spoonful with enough batter to make a tiny dumpling. Drop into batter and fry.

CAULIFLOWER

Tear off flowerettes of cauliflower, salt them, dust with flour, dip in batter and drop in deep oil. Also use the leaves and root; very tasty.

BURDOCK ROOT

This is the toughest of the root vegetables and will require precooking. Sauté with a little water for twenty minutes to a half hour. Mix slivers of precooked burdock and slivers of carrot. Dip a spoonful into batter and drop in oil.

CELERY

Chop celery very fine and use in combination with onions or carrots. Dip in batter and then drop into hot oil.

BROCCOLI

Handle exactly like cauliflower. Break into flowerettes, dip in batter and fry in oil.

CORN

Scrape the kernels off an ear of corn and mix with chopped onion. Stir in a spoonful of batter to make a tiny dumpling, and fry in deep oil.

CHESTNUTS

See the recipe for chestnut croquettes, which is nothing but a fancied-up version of tempura.

CLAMS

Fried clams have been a specialty of Howard Johnson's restaurants for years. Clams are usually steamed to make them easier to open. Use the residual liquor to make the tempura batter—as detailed in the recipe for mussels tempura. Dust the clams with flour, dip them in a batter made of buckwheat or whole wheat flour and deep fry.

EGGS

This is tricky, but the result has eggs benedict beat a mile. Prepare 1 egg at a time, using only fertilized eggs from organically fed hens. (If you have been on a macrobiotic diet for a while and eat a nonfertilized egg, don't be surprised if you get a rash all over your chest and back.)

Pour a small amount of tempura batter into a small bowl. Break an egg into the batter, and cover the egg with the batter. Then gently slide the egg and the batter into the hot oil. For egg tempura, the oil should not be as hot as usual—just hot enough to cook the batter without hard-boiling the egg. When the batter has cooked firm and slightly golden, remove from the pan and serve pronto.

FISH

Almost any fish filet can be done up as a tempura. Cut the filets into 2-inch squares, dust with flour and salt, then dip in batter and fry.

LOTUS ROOT

Most macrobiotic restaurants serve lotus root tempura without batter. They cut the lotus root into thin slices, salt them well and allow to drain for an hour, then fry the slices naked in deep oil.

ONIONS

Onions are great as an added ingredient to any mixture of vegetables for tempura. They are also great on their own. Here are two ways to handle them.

The first is the conventional onion rings: Slice the onion in rounds, dust the rings with flour, dip in batter and fry.

The other way is to cut the onions in half lengthwise, slicing them thin, leaving the hard root at the bottom intact to hold the slivers together. Spread this piece of vegetable sculpture out like a fan, dust with flour, dip in batter and deep fry.

OYSTERS

Opening oysters without getting fragments of shell all over them is the toughest part. It is easier to work with pre-opened oysters by the pint. Reserve the liquor and use it in your tempura batter instead of water. Shake the oysters in a paper sack with a few tablespoons of flour, then dip in batter and deep fry.

PARSNIPS

Tempura turns this lowly vegetable into a near-dessert. You can sliver the parsnips like carrots, and spoon into the batter. Or you can cut them into long thin strips like julienne potatoes, shake them in a sack of flour, dip in batter and fry.

PUMPKINS

Pumpkin is best handled in not-so-small slices, dipped in salt and flour and then in batter.

SCALLOPS

Salt them and let them stand for a while. Then dust them with flour, dip in batter and deep fry.

SHRIMP

Easy to handle. Peel and clean the shrimp. Boil the shells in water, salted to taste, to make a stock. Cool the stock and use it in the tempura batter instead of water. Salt the shrimp and let them stand a bit. Then shake them in a paper sack with a few tablespoons flour. Cornmeal is great with shrimp. Dip in batter and deep fry.

TURNIPS

Handle the same way as parsnips.

WATERCRESS

There are two ways to handle watercress: the first is to take a full stalk of watercress, dust it with flour, dip in batter and drop in oil. The other way is to chop the watercress into 1-inch pieces, and spoon them into the batter like slivered carrots.

ZUCCHINI

Start by not peeling this or any other vegetable. Cut it up into long thin strips or halves and cut into 1-inch slices. Dust with flour in a paper sack, dip in batter and fry.

Serve all tempura as hot as you can manage, with a tiny bit of grated raw white radish on the side, served in small individual bowls about the size of a teacup, and with the precious soy sauce handy enough so that each piece may be dunked.

FISH KEBBAB

This is the fanciest and it seems tastiest form of tempura. It has had a great success at many restaurants. Serve it to guests, or simply to your husband, accompanied with rice and a tiny bit of salad. It's delicious.

Buy wooden skewers at Japanese stores. Cut the vegetables into large thin pieces. Carrots, for instance, should be cut very thin, otherwise they will not cook through. Put three or four cabbage leaves together and cut them into 1-inch squares. Cut pepper (yin) vertically into 8 parts, and then cut crosswise into two parts. Break cauliflower into its flowerlets and slice the stem part. Thread onto the skewers in this order: onion, pepper, carrot, cauliflower and onion again, etc.

Fish is even easier to handle. Use preferably filet of sole or filet of flounder and skewer it alternately with the vegetables. Dust with flour, immerse in tempura batter and deep fry in oil 3/4 inch deep.

About eating only rice

"Should a person, to gain total freedom, eat only rice?" The young man who asked the question had already asked it three times during the past two years.

"A free person can eat anything, and it will not do him any harm. Still, yes, eating only rice will give him total freedom. But you live here in a city, and the air is bad, everything is very bad, like the vegetables which are chemically grown. Ideally, one should live on rice, in the mountains, in healthful air. However, one should never eat only rice without consulting me or some friends who know about it. You must eat and enjoy food. To eat only rice is a big decision."

Hors d'oeuvres and accompaniments

VEGETABLE PATE

Made out of vegetables and bread, this pâté tastes like liver pâté. One can hardly notice the difference. It has been a tremendous and increasing success among vegetarians and even meat-eater friends. Cook it for fun! If you fail, buy next door a real liver pâté and tell your guests it's made of vegetables; they'll believe you! But try again, you will succeed.

Hors d'oeuvres and accompaniments « 79

Here is what you need:

>2 onions
>2 cups cooked lentils
>1/2 pound yeasted bread
>1 tablespoon oil
>pinch thyme
>pinch coriander
>pinch nutmeg
>1 or 2 bay leaves
>1/2 teaspoon salt
>1 tablespoon sesame butter
>1 tablespoon miso
>3 tablespoons parsley, chopped

Sauté the onions in the oil, stirring, until they turn golden. (10 minutes, medium flame.) Throw in moist bread, prepared ahead by soaking for at least 1 hour in water and then pressing to remove excess moisture. Keep stirring the mixture, adding water as necessary. Cook for 15 minutes over a medium flame. Add thyme, bayleaf, coriander, nutmeg, salt and parsley. Stir 5 more minutes. Add lentils (previously cooked and blended in a mixer) and stir again. The mixture should be very heavy. Add miso, sesame butter and stir 5 more minutes. Pour the whole mixture in a mold and put in the oven. Bake 30 minutes at 325°. Serve cool or lukewarm.

PURÉE DE LENTILLES

This spread keeps in the refrigerator for a few days.

        1 cup lentils
        1/2 tablespoon miso
        1 pinch nutmeg
        2 tablespoons parsley
        salt to taste

Cook the lentils. Some water should remain. Purée in blender. The purée should be thick. Add the miso, nutmeg, parsley and salt. Cook without covering for 15 minutes over a low flame. Serve warm or cool.

CROQUETTES DE LENTILLES

        2 cups lentils
        4 tablespoons whole wheat flour
        1 small onion finely chopped
        1 tablespoon parsley
        salt to taste

Cook the lentils, retaining the water. Blend in a vegetable mill; the mixture comes out very thick. Add the raw onion, parsley and salt. Stir in flour. Roll the mixture into small balls (about 1 tablespoon to a ball). Fry in a frying pan with just enough corn oil to cover the bottom of the pan.

THE CAVIAR OF THE POOR
(Fish-roe spread)

> 3 to 4 ounces roe
> 2 tablespoons sesame butter
> 1 tablespoon soya sauce
> 1 to 2 tablespoons water

Boil the roe in boiling water for 10 minutes. Remove the skin. Blend roe, sesame butter, soya sauce and water in mixer. Serve cool. Could also be prepared by stirring all ingredients rather than blending in mixer.

CROQUETTES OF CHICK PEAS

> 2 cups chick peas
> 4 tablespoons whole wheat flour
> 1/2 clove garlic, finely chopped
> 1 tablespoon parsley
> salt to taste

Cook the chick peas until soft. The fastest way is to let them soak over night and then cook them 1-1/2 hours with dashi kombu (this seaweed helps to soften any hard vegetable; 1 piece 3 x 3 inches is enough). Crush the peas with a fork after you have poured off some water. The chick peas should be wet enough to enable you to crush them easily. Add the garlic, parsley, whole wheat flour and salt. Mix very well. Toss little balls into a frying pan with a tablespoon. Height of the oil in the frying pan: 1/4 inch.

MIDDLE EASTERN *MEZE*
HUMMUS TAHINA

The Middle Eastern meze *is the Arabic answer to the French hors d'oeuvres, an opening gambit to a festive meal. The Arabs were dipping fingers into spicy concoctions centuries before cocktail party and barbecue pit hostesses began making party dips out of ersatz soups and processed cheeses. The ideal dip for this adaptation of a traditional Middle Eastern* meze *is a hunk of dark bread or a rice cake. If you insist on neatness, keep hot wet towels or fingerbowls on hand for the finger-tip dippers.*

>   1/2 pound chick peas
>   olive oil
>   1 cup tahini
>   2 or 3 cloves garlic, crushed
>   1 cup water
>   2 tablespoons mint leaves, fresh or dried,
>   finely chopped
>   sea salt as needed

Cook the chick peas slowly in plenty of water, for about 4 hours until they are soft and can be put through a food mill or blender. They should have the consistency of a fine paste. Add the crushed garlic, stir in the tahini, the oil and the salt. Thin the mixture with water to the consistency of a sturdy mayonnaise. Stir in the mint. Serve in a large shallow dish or individual saucers. If the mixture is too thick, add a little more water. (This recipe will produce enough for a sizable group and can be cut down as desired.) Dip bread—or fingers—into the paste and savor the flavor. To fortify the mixture, a spoonful of miso will give it a real protein kick.

CRESSON SUR CANAPE
(Watercress on the couch)

It's French. It seems as if the very green vegetable is inviting you for a minute of love; not that it takes a minute to chew a canape!

> 1 bunch watercress
> 4 large, thin slices yeasted bread
> 2 tablespoons sesame oil
> soy sauce
> salt to taste

Sauté (about 15 minutes) the watercress in 1 tablespoon of sesame oil. Add salt. Moisten the bread slightly with water—the most practical is to sprinkle water on the bread with your hands. Heat a frying pan, oil it with remaining sesame oil and toast the bread for 5 minutes on each side. The flame should not be too high.

Serve the watercress on the bread, adding some soy sauce. Important: both bread and watercress must be served hot.

FRITES

This is our potato chip. It has an advantage: it's not made out of potato but out of cornmeal.

>2 cups cornmeal
>1 cup white flour
>water
>salt

Knead the cornmeal and flour with water, adding very slowly; the dough should not stick or be too dry. Roll the dough very thin. Cut in the form you want, square or round. The pieces should not be bigger than 1-1/2 inches. Preheat your oil, and toss the pieces of dough into it. A golden color indicates that they are ready to be picked up. As in any deep frying process, drain them on paper napkins to absorb the excess oil. Sprinkle salt according to taste.

BUCKWHEAT CHIPS

Same process as for corn chips.

>2 cups buckwheat flour
>1 cup white flour

KARINTO

These could be described as deep-fried cookies. But artful blending and changing the kinds of flour used, and varying the small amounts of accessories—nuts, peanuts, raisins, grated orange rind and roasted sesame seed—will make you forget that karinto have no unnatural sweetening. After buckwheat, corn seems sugared. It's all relative—yin and yang.

    2 cups flour
    2 tablespoons sesame seeds
    1 teaspoon cinnamon
    salt
    water

Mix the dry ingredients thoroughly, then knead with enough water to form a soft dough. Keep kneading for a good 10 minutes. Roll the dough out thin and cut into any shape that appeals to you. Fry in deep oil until crisp.

Buckwheat flour seems best with just sesame seeds, at least to some palates.

Minced dried orange peel works great with millet flour.

If you want to prepare this simply, roll the dough into a sausage shape and fry the slices.

MISO SPREAD

Fast and easy to make when you suddenly have a group of hungry friends home! Put in front of them a loaf of bread and a bowl of spread. They'll stuff themselves.

    1 tablespoonful miso
    4 tablespoonfuls sesame butter
    1 or 2 tablespoons water
    1 teaspoon minced orange peel

Mix miso, sesame butter and water. Cook 5 minutes while stirring. Some water will evaporate and the mixture will thicken. When cooked, mix in minced orange peel.

VARIATION

This second version is even more economical; there is flour and more water in it!

    3 tablespoonfuls sesame butter
    1 tablespoonful miso
    1 tablespoonful oat flour
    1/2 cup water
    basil or mint, a pinch

Cook the sesame butter in a saucepan while stirring until golden. Add the miso and keep stirring. Add the oat flour diluted in 1/2 cup water and pour it on the blended miso and sesame butter. Add either basil or mint. Stir. Leave the saucepan uncovered and cook 15 minutes, stirring constantly.

MISO-ONION SPREAD

    1 tablespoon miso
    1/4 onion
    4 tablespoons water
    2 tablespoons parsley, finely chopped

Dilute the miso with the water. Add the chopped onion and parsley. Mix well.

MISO IN GREEN

    1 tablespoon miso
    1/4 fresh pepper
    4 tablespoons water
    1 scallion

Burn the skin of a pepper evenly by turning it slowly over a flame. This takes 10 to 15 minutes over a medium flame. Remove the blackened skin under running water. Chop 1/4 of the pepper finely. Cut the scallion into tiny pieces. Dilute the miso with the water and stir in the other ingredients.

Very good for sandwiches.

SPREAD OF SARDINES

    1 can sardines
    3 tablespoons sesame butter
    2 tablespoons soya sauce
    2 tablespoons water

Buy a can of sardines packed with pure olive oil, if possible from a health food store. Take out the bones and crush them. Add the sesame butter, soya sauce and water. Mix well. Serve on thin slices of bread.

ENDIVES ON THE BEACH

    4 cups cooked rice
    1 pound endives
    2 small apples
    1 dozen walnuts
    3 tablespoons olive or corn oil
    5 tablespoons umeboshi juice

If the rice is sticky, this salad will not have the proper texture. Rinse rice under cold water and let drain completely. Wash the endive and cut into pieces. Slice the apples. Mix the umeboshi juice and corn or olive oil. Pour over rice in a salad bowl. Mix and turn delicately before serving.

SALADE D'ENDIVES

Cut 2 endives into 1/2-inch pieces and mix them with a dozen olives. Make a sauce of umeboshi juice, olive oil and soy sauce (*see* Sauces) and pour it on the salad. In hot summer, add two or three slices of orange.

SUMMERTIME

This is Lima's (George Ohsawa's wife) recipe. You can't miss, it is delicious.

> 3 onions
> 2 stalks celery
> 2 carrots, medium size
> 5 cabbage leaves
> 1 turnip (white)
> 2 apples
> 1 egg
> 1/2 pound dandelion leaves, chopped
> 4 lettuce leaves
> watercress for garnish
> salt
>
> Dressing:
> 5 tablespoons oil
> 3 teaspoons salt
> juice of orange

Chop finely the onions and celery stalks. Cut the carrots into matchstick-size pieces and boil in a small amount of water for 2 minutes; drain in a strainer. Shred the cabbage leaves and soak them one or two minutes in boiling water. Cut the turnips into matchstick-size pieces and sprinkle with salt; after 10 minutes, press to remove juice. Cut apples in thin pieces and sprinkle lightly with salt. Boil the egg. Mix the oil with 3 teaspoons of salt and add the juice of an orange. Combine the onion, celery, turnip, cabbage, carrot and chopped dandelion leaves. Put in a dish lined with lettuce leaves and garnish with watercress. Pour on dressing. Grate the hard-boiled egg on the top.

About balance

There were 70 persons around him that day. The sun was shining through the open windows. Everyone was happy; the Master had just finished saying that he had never received such good answers since he had left Japan.

The lecture that afternoon was more philosophical than anything else. The Master was happy about it; at last no question about food. An old lady, however, spoiled it all: "Mister Ohsawa, once in a while I have to go out and eat with some friends; so I am compelled to eat some animal food. How, for example, would you balance a piece of beef?"

The Master smiled. One or two disciples turned their heads toward the spoiler. Beef!!!

The lady continued: "Would it be possible to balance it with salad or with a glass of wine?"

Ohsawa again took his time in answering: "Some animal foods are very difficult to balance, like regular cheese, beef, etc. They are yin because of too much acidity and toxins. Others such as goat cheese, lamb, bird, fish and grain can be balanced more easily with raw or cooked vegetables or even fruits. It is as though you asked me if one could balance an elephant with a crocodile. It is better to avoid eating beef than think to balance it, because there is nothing to balance it; it is beef!! and very bad! French people balance a piece of goat cheese with a little bit of wine . . . very good judgment! One should never force the balance of a meal. You do not, for instance, force a man and a woman into marriage. Give them first a chance to know and sympathize with each other."

Soups

And God said, Behold, I have given you every herb bearing seed, which is upon the face of all the earth, and every tree, in which is the fruit of a tree yielding seed; to you it shall be for meat. GENESIS 1:29

PUMPKIN SOUP

The lovely lowly pumpkin has practically vanished from the American urban scene except as a Hallowe'en prop for children or as a base for a pie made—if at all—out of a can. But pumpkin is much too yang and too delicious to be ignored by any macrobiotic cook. Pumpkin soup sounds like the oddest dish of all but one try will certainly make it a permanent fixture on your winter menu.

        pumpkin
        onion, finely chopped
        oil
        sea salt
        flour (whole wheat)

Use the smallest amount of oil possible to sauté the finely chopped onion and cut-up pumpkin. Proportions can be adjusted to suit your taste: usually 1 pound of pumpkin to a good-sized onion. Use the skin of both pumpkin and onions. After sautéing the vegetables, add enough water to cover. Boil slowly until the pumpkin falls apart. Salt to taste. Strain or put through a vegetable mill. Brown a small amount of flour in vegetable oil, mix with water enough to make a thin paste. Blend this into the pumpkin mixture and boil again slowly.

Serve with toasted bread croutons, shredded parsley. Sometimes the pumpkin mixture turns out to be thick enough to serve without adding the flour mixture. In that case, make small dumplings out of flour, salt and water, add them to the pumpkin mixture 30 to 40 minutes before serving. Buckwheat dumplings, whole wheat dumplings, or a mixture of several kinds of flour may be used. Almost anything goes with this staple dish.

The Hokkaido pumpkin from northern Japan has a taste much closer to the American squash, which may also be used as a basis for soup. Carrots can also be used in the same way as pumpkin to make a delicious soup—or blend the two. The soup works in almost any ratio of these vegetables.

VARIATION (for 6 persons)

2 onions, medium size
1 pound pumpkin
1 cup semolina
croutons
parsley
sea salt
1 tablespoon sesame oil for the semolina
1 tablespoon sesame oil for the vegetables

Roast the semolina in oil in a pan. Sauté the vegetables in oil. Add 1/2 cup water and salt. Time for the nituke: over a high flame 5 minutes; add water, 15 minutes over low flame. Purée the vegetables in the blender. Pour the mixture and roasted semolina into six to eight cups of boiling water. Cook 15 minutes more and add salt. The soup should be heavy. Serve with croutons and parsley.

You can also make this soup with oatmeal or without any flour at all.

SOUP OF OAT FLAKES
(for 6 persons)

>4 onions, small, cut into small moons
>1 cup oat flakes, slightly roasted in pan
>sea salt
>1 tablespoon corn oil
>soy sauce

Heat the oil in a frying pan. Cook the onions in the oil over a high flame for 3 to 5 minutes, stirring, and over a low flame 8 to 10 minutes. Onions should be golden in color. Pour the onions, flakes and salt into six to eight cups boiling water. Stir. Cook on low flame for 20 to 25 minutes. Add soya sauce before serving. Stir again.

GARDEN RICE SOUP
(for 6 persons)

>4 tablespoons roasted rice cream (very fine)
>1 tablespoon sunflower oil
>1 onion, large
>1 scallion
>1 carrot, large
>1 turnip, small
>1 stalk celery
>salt to taste

Gradually stir the roasted rice cream into 6 cups of cold water. Stirring constantly, slowly bring to a boil, then reduce the flame. Cook on very low flame for 15 minutes. Sauté onion, scallion, carrot and turnip in oil. Add 1 cup of water, salt and celery. Cook on low flame for 15 minutes. Pour rice cream and vegetables into six to eight cups boiling water. Pour into a blender, blend and then return to pot. Cook on low flame for 15 minutes.

SEMOULINETTE
(for 6 persons)

> 1 cup wheat semolina
> 1 clove garlic, finely chopped
> 2 bay leaves
> sea salt
> 8 cups boiling water
> 1 tablespoon olive or sesame oil

Roast the semolina in oil until golden. Add to the boiling water. Add salt, bay leaves and garlic. Cook 5 minutes over high flame, stirring constantly. Cook an additional 25 minutes over a low flame, stirring frequently.

The wheat semolina can be bought at any Armenian store. If you do not like the garlic, for one reason or another, use only bay leaf.

BARLEY SOUP (for 6 persons)

6 tablespoons barley flour
8 cups boiling water
1 tablespoon sesame butter
1 tablespoon sesame oil
croutons
parsley

Roast the flour slightly in heated sesame oil until golden. Using a wooden spoon, stir the roasted flour into boiling water. Add salt. Cook on low flame for 10 minutes. Soup should be heavy but not thick. Do not forget to stir constantly. Add sesame butter and cook another 10 minutes. Serve with croutons and parsley.

MISO SOUP (for 6 persons)

Miso soup is inseparable from traditional Japanese life. Miso is a pasty seasoning made from fermented soybeans and malted wheat; various kinds are made in Japan, depending on the locality. A wide variety of miso soup can be made by putting different ingredients together. In winter macrobiotic friends cook it at least twice a week. If you feel weak, here is your pep pill!

2 onions, small, finely chopped
3 carrots, finely chopped
2 strips of dried wakame
3 or 4 cabbage leaves
6 to 8 cups boiling water
1-1/2 tablespoons miso
1 tablespoon corn oil

Sauté the vegetables in the corn oil: 5 minutes over high flame, then 5 minutes over a low flame. Pour the sautéed vegetables into the boiling water. Add in sliced wakame. Add the miso, diluted in 1/2 cup water. Cook over low flame for 15 minutes. You may add cooked whole wheat noodles just before the end.

CLEAR RIVER (for 6 persons)

It takes time to cook, but not to prepare!

>   2 carrots
>   6 onions, very small
>   2 stalks celery
>   1 fresh burdock root
>   1/4 teaspoon ginger
>   soy sauce
>   sea salt

It is much better not to cut the onions; just remove their skins. If you do not like onions, use turnips. Cut the vegetables into big pieces. Add the vegetables to boiling water. Add a little bit of salt. Cook over low flame for 30 minutes. Add ginger and soy sauce. Cook over low flame for 20 minutes.

WATERCRESS SOUP (for 6 persons)

>   1 cup wheat semolina
>   2 handfuls watercress, chopped
>   1 tablespoon sesame oil
>   sea salt
>   croutons

Roast the semolina in oil in a pan. Sprinkle carefully over boiling water, stirring at the same time. Add salt. Cook 30 minutes over low flame. Add the watercress. Serve with croutons.

Before adding the watercress you can blend the soup. This will give to it a "veloute."

VERMICELLI SOUP
(for 4 persons)

    1 cup of vermicelli
    1 tablespoon kuzu or arrowroot
    soy sauce
    parsley
    sea salt
    7 to 9 cups of water

Dilute the arrowroot in a cup of cold water. Add diluted arrowroot to 6 to 8 cups of boiling water, stirring constantly. Add the vermicelli and salt. Cook on low flame for 10 minutes. Add soy sauce. Cook on low flame for 5 minutes. Add parsley before serving.

VARIATION (for 6 persons)

    2 scallions
    1 stalk celery
    2 carrots
    1 turnip
    8 to 10 cups water
    1 tablespoon sesame oil
    sea salt
    soy sauce
    1-1/2 pounds vermicelli

Chop the vegetables. Sauté in oil, using high flame for 5 minutes, and a low flame for 10 minutes. Add the vegetables and salt to boiling water. Stirring, cook on low flame for 20 minutes. Add the vermicelli. Cook on low flame for 5 minutes. Add soy sauce. Stir!

CARROT SOUP (for 6 persons)

      1 onion, large, chopped
      3 or 4 carrots, chopped
      5 tablespoons whole wheat flour
      1 pinch thyme
      1 bay leaf
      1 tablespoon corn oil for vegetables
      1 tablespoon corn oil for flour
      croutons
      sea salt
      6 to 8 cups boiling water

Saute carrots and onion in oil. Mix the vegetables with some water and blend in a mixer. Brown the flour in oil until the color is golden. Add the roasted flour and the blended vegetables to boiling water. Add salt, thyme and bay leaf. Cook over low flame for 30 minutes. Serve with croutons.

CHINESE SOUP
(for 6 persons)

    1 strip dried wakame
    2 onions, medium size, sliced
    3 turnips, very small, sliced
    6 cups boiling water
    1 tablespoon miso
    3 tablespoons whole wheat flour, roasted
    1 tablespoon arrowroot
    1 tablespoon corn oil
    sea salt
    croutons

Boil the vegetables with the wakame. Add the whole wheat flour. Cook on low flame for 25 minutes. Dissolve the arrowroot in 1/2 cup water. Mix in a blender the cooked vegetables, arrow root and miso. Add salt and boiling water. Cook on low flame for 10 minutes more. Serve with croutons.

SCALLION SOUP
(for 6 persons)

    1 onion, medium size, cut into thin moons
    3 to 4 scallions with greens, finely chopped
    3 tablespoons oatmeal
    6 to 8 cups boiling water
    1 tablespoon corn oil
    sea salt

Saute onions and scallions for no more than 5 minutes over high flame. Add 1/2 cup water and salt. Cook 15 minutes on low flame. Pour into boiling water. Add the oatmeal previously roasted or oat flakes as they are. Cook 30 minutes over low flame. Add scallions and onions.

FRESH CORN ON A GREEN FIELD (for 6 persons)

    2 corn on the cob
    1 onion, large
    1 strip dried wakame
    2 tablespoons fresh green peas
    2 stalks celery, with leaves
    6 cups boiling water
    1 teaspoon corn oil
    1 tablespoon arrowroot
    sea salt
    parsley

Cut kernels off corncobs. Sauté the onion in corn oil over high flame for 5 minutes. To boiling water, add the corn grains removed from the cob, wakame, green peas, celery. Add the arrowroot diluted in 1/2 cup cold water. Add salt. Cook over low flame for 40 minutes. Salt according to taste. Sprinkle with parsley to serve.

POLENTA SOUP
(for 8 persons)

> 1 cup polenta
> 2 onions, large, finely chopped
> 2 carrots, finely chopped
> 4 scallions, finely chopped
> 1 turnip, small, finely chopped
> 1/4 teaspoon thyme
> 1 tablespoon corn oil for polenta
> 1 tablespoon corn oil for vegetables
> 10 to 12 cups water

Slightly roast the polenta in corn oil in a pan until the yellow color turns to light brown. For a uniform color, stir. This should not take more than 10 minutes. Sauté the vegetables. To 10 to 12 cups boiling water, add the polenta, vegetables, salt and thyme. Cook over low flame for 50 minutes.

You can buy the polenta at any Italian store.

MILLET SOUP
(for 6 to 8 persons)

> 2 onions, medium size, finely chopped
> 1/4 cabbage head, finely chopped
> 2 carrots, finely chopped
> 6 to 8 cups water
> 1 cup millet
> 1 tablespoon corn oil
> sea salt
> 2 bay leaves
> thyme—a pinch

Sauté the vegetables in corn oil. Roast the millet for 10 minutes. Pour vegetables and millet into boiling water. Add salt, thyme and bay leaves. Cook over low flame for 50 minutes. Keep pot covered while the soup is cooking. It is the one necessary secret for better taste.

LA BELLE JARDINIERE
(for 8 persons)

    1 cup azuki beans
    1/2 cup oat flakes
    2 stalks celery, finely chopped
    1 pinch coriander
    1 pinch thyme
    8 to 10 cups water
    2 bay leaves
    1 tablespoon miso
    1 tablespoon sesame butter (tahini)
    sea salt

Soak the azuki beans overnight. Drain water. Add the azuki and some salt to boiling water. Cook over medium flame for 45 minutes, stirring frequently. Add the celery, oat flakes, miso, tahini, coriander and thyme. Reduce the flame and cook for another 45 minutes. Do not forget to cover and stir!

POTIRON-POIS CHICHE
(Pumpkin-chick peas)
(for 6 to 8 persons)

1-1/2 cup chick peas
1-1/2 pounds pumpkin (with skin)
1 cup oat flakes
1/4 teaspoon thyme or cumin
1 tablespoon olive oil
1 clove garlic (optional)
sea salt
10-1/2 cups water

Soak the chick peas overnight. Drain. Sauté the pumpkin in olive oil, then cook 15 minutes with 1/2 cup water. Cook the chick peas in approximately 10 cups of water, for 40 minutes, covered, over a low flame. Spoon out chick peas. Mix the chick peas and sautéed pumpkin in a blender. Pour this mixture into water in which the chick peas were cooked. Add thyme, oat flakes, salt and, if you wish, crushed garlic. Cook 25 minutes longer on a low, low flame, stirring. Soup should be heavy, almost like a cream, but still liquid! This soup could be made without the pumpkin.

SOUPE AUX LENTILLES
(for 6 persons)

>1 cup of lentils
3/4 cup oat flakes
2 handfuls stale bread
1 pinch thyme
1 bay leaf
sea salt
parsley, chopped
5 to 6 cups water

Soak the lentils overnight. Drain and cook them in 4 to 5 cups of water for 40 minutes over a low flame. Mix them in a blender. To 5 to 6 cups boiling water, add lentils, bread cut in pieces, thyme, bay leaf and salt. Cook the mixture 20 minutes more on a very low flame. Serve with chopped parsley. The soup should be heavy.

KOI-KOKU

The most advanced "pep pills," "bennies" and all the modern recipes for quick energy builders hardly hold a candle to this ancient Japanese dish. Dancers and athletes find it habit-forming. They want it before each performance or competition. It is also good for inflammations, including inflammations of the middle ear; pneumonia, arthritis and rheumatism and fever. It is also recommended for nursing mothers with insufficient milk. In that case, the entire dish should be taken over a 5-day period. Koi-koku is based on one of the most yin among fish and the most yang of vegetables: carp and burdock.

>carp, small
>burdock roots, 3 times the amount of fish
>3 heaping tablespoons miso
>sesame oil
>used bancha tea leaves

A good fish market in a Jewish neighborhood is the best place to find a live carp. Ask the man to fish out a small one from the tank and to remove only the gall bladder. Some of the other customers may look at you strangely, but chances are the man behind the counter will take it in stride—he's had the same request before.

Cut the fish into 1/2-inch slices, using head, scales, fins, everything.

Shred the burdock roots like shavings when you sharpen a pencil. Then sauté them in a small amount of oil. Put the carp slices on top and add enough water to cover.

Tie a cupful of used leaves of bancha tea in a small sack of cheesecloth and drop them on top of the fish. Simmer this mixture for at least 3 hours and as long as 12. If the water evaporates, add more little by little. The carp—head, bones and all—will have completely disintegrated while the hardy burdock shavings are still intact.

When the fish has disintegrated, take out the tea leaves, and add the miso after thinning it with a little water. Then let the soup simmer another hour or more.

If you have a pressure cooker, you can cook the soup 2 hours under pressure and continue cooking without pressure.

Then fasten your seatbelt and eat everything—even the vestiges of bones. The taste, needless to say, seems wild and gamy on the first round but you haven't lived until you've tried it.

AZUKI SOUP (for 8 persons)

Do not be discouraged by the time it takes to make a soup as good as this! By cooking you will develop ability and patience.

> 3 pieces, 3 inches long, kombu
> 1 cup azuki beans
> 3/4 cup oat flakes
> 1 onion, finely chopped
> 1 tablespoon sesame oil
> croutons
> sea salt
> parsley
> 8 cups water

Soak the azuki overnight in lukewarm water. Drain and cook in 8 cups of water with the kombu. Cook for 50 minutes on low flame after bringing to a boil. Add salt and cook 10 minutes longer. Sauté the onion. Mix everything in the blender. Pour the mixture into boiling water. Add the oat flakes and salt. Cook 30 minutes on low flame. Serve with croutons and parsley.

The kombu helps the azuki cook faster.

CAULIFLOWER SOUP
(for 8 persons)

    2 carrots, small
    1 onion, large
    2 pounds cauliflower
    1/2 cup whole wheat flour
    2 tablespoons corn oil for flour
    1 tablespoon corn oil for vegetables
    sea salt

Sauté the vegetables in the corn oil for 10 minutes over a high flame. Add 1/2 cup of water and salt. Cook 10 minutes over a low flame. Roast the whole wheat flour in a pan until it is golden in color. Add vegetables and flour to boiling water. Add salt. Cook 1 hour over a low flame.

SOUP OF FRESH NOODLES
(for 6 persons)

This takes time only because of the preparation of the noodles.

> 4 onions, small, finely chopped
> 1 tablespoon corn oil
> 6 to 8 cups water
> 1 cup whole wheat flour
> 1 cup unbleached flour
> sea salt

Sauté the onions. Make a dough of the two flours and a little water. Flatten it as thin as possible and cut it into 1-inch square pieces. To boiling water, add the noodles first and then onions and salt. Cook for 20 minutes over a low flame.

You may sprinkle soup with swiss cheese when you serve it or sprinkle grated swiss cheese into each bowl, and place under broiler for 10 minutes. Remove when the cheese gets brownish.

MUSSEL SOUP
(for 6 to 8 persons)

Mussels, like oysters, clams, shrimp and other shellfish, "do not run away." While less yang than shrimp, they are less yin than oysters. Also they are plentiful in most seacoast areas, which also means they are inexpensive. Properly handled, the lowly mussel can be as delectable as expensive shrimps or oysters. A simple soup of mussels is easy to make and delicious.

>   40 to 50 mussels
>   2 onions, small, diced
>   1/2 cup white wine
>   1 clove garlic, minced
>   1 tablespoon olive oil
>   sea salt
>   parsley

Scrub the mussels thoroughly in cold water. Sauté the onions in olive oil. Place the scrubbed mussels on the bottom of the pot. Add the wine and a small amount of water. Boil over a medium heat until the steam opens the shells; then add a dash of salt and boil some more. The soup is ready to serve when the mussels are practically free of their shells. Add parsley 5 minutes before steaming is complete—when some mussels pull free of shells.

SOUPE AUX CHOUX (CABBAGE SOUP) (for 6 persons)

    1 cabbage
    2 tablespoons sesame butter
    12 thin slices of bread
    sea salt

Boil nearly 2 quarts of water. Cut the cabbage into 4 parts and put it in the boiling water. Add salt. Cook over low flame for 1 hour and 30 minutes. Add the sesame butter and stir. Pour over 2 slices of bread for each serving.

SOUPE QUARTIER LATIN (for 6 persons)

    2 carrots
    2 turnips
    2 stalks celery
    2 scallions
    3 onions
    1 pound pumpkin
    1 bunch parsley
    saffron
    sea salt

Cut the vegetables and boil them in about 2 quarts of salty water for 40 minutes. Strain through a colander. Add saffron and salt. Return to the fire for 20 minutes, stirring. Soup is ready to serve.

PUMPKIN AND BEAN SOUP
(for 8 persons)

        1/2 pound azuki beans
        1/2 pound pumpkin (Japanese), chopped
        1 small cabbage
        8 cups water
        3 onions, small, sliced
        sea salt
        coriander
        nutmeg
        2 tablespoons sesame oil

Soak azuki beans overnight; drain. Sauté the onions in oil. Add the pumpkin. Sauté for 15 to 20 minutes over medium flame. Pour the mixture into a pot. Add water, salt, cabbage, azuki beans, coriander and nutmeg. Cook covered at least 2 hours over low flame.

ONION SOUP
(for 6 to 8 persons)

Do not be frightened by the cooking time. This soup is one of the best, and besides it does not require much work.

> 2 onions, thinly sliced
> 3/4 cup whole wheat flour
> sea salt
> 1 tablespoon corn oil for onions
> 1 tablespoon corn oil to roast the whole wheat flour
> croutons

Sauté the onions. Roast the flour in a pan until it is golden. Pour onions and flour into boiling water, stirring. Cook over a low flame for 1 hour to 1 hour and 20 minutes. Serve with croutons (optional).

This soup is good when cooked very long. Do not forget to stir from time to time and to keep pot covered.

FRENCH ONION SOUP

Tamari is the secret ingredient of this delicious and foolproof onion soup. It is easy to double the quantities and use half the stock—without the tamari—instead of water in making buckwheat cream the following day. The quantity of onions in relation to water depends entirely on the size of the onions, so use your own judgment.

    onions, finely chopped
    sea salt
    water
    tamari
    oil

Cut the onions very fine—use outer skins as well, that's where that strong French color comes from. Sauté the onions in a small amount of oil. Add water and simmer slowly until done —usually about an hour. Add sea salt and tamari, simmer another 5 minutes and serve steaming hot, with toasted bread or croutons.

The soup may be served hot, letting each individual add tamari according to his taste. It may also be put through a vegetable mill or blender before adding the tamari.

PURÉED TURNIP SOUP
(for 6 persons)

       2 lbs turnips, cut
       2 tablespoons whole wheat flour
       2 tablespoons olive oil
       sea salt
       1 pinch nutmeg
       6 cups water

Heat the oil. Add the flour and stir until it becomes golden in color. Add the turnips. Add the water, salt and nutmeg. Cook for 1/2 hour over a low flame. Mix in a blender. Place again on the fire for a few minutes.

LA SOUPE DE PROVENCE
(for 10 to 12 persons)

In Provence the sun shines almost all the year round. People are happy. Sometimes we wonder if it's the soup that made them so or if it's the contrary. Nevertheless one cannot succeed in making this soup and being sad.

>5 ounces scallions, finely chopped
>5 ounces carrots, finely chopped
>1-1/2 pounds sea fish: red snapper, sole, etc.
>4 ounces vermicelli
>4 tablespoons olive oil
>2 cloves garlic
>1 pinch saffron, diluted in water
>1 red pepper
>3 to 4 cups water

Sauté the garlic first in olive oil in a saucepan. Add the scallions and carrots. Add any kind of fish that has been washed and cleaned. Add 3 or 4 cups of water and saffron. Add salt. Cover and cook for 40 minutes over a medium flame. Remove bones from fish. Pound the vegetables and fish. Return to fire. Add vermicelli and let soup cook for another 10 minutes.

LA BOUILLABAISSE!
(for 12 persons)

If a Marseillais tells you the bouillabaisse of Marseilles is the best in the world, believe him. The most important ingredient in making bouillabaisse is your own happy spirit.

There is a song that gives the secret of how to succeed to make a good one:

> "To make a good bouillabaisse
> One must rise early in the morning,
> Prepare a pastis for one's friends,
> Telling them stories with one's hands.
> Ah! How good is a bouillabaise!
> Ah! My God how good it is!"

3 pounds of fish: sole, whiting, mackerel, red snapper, mussels
6 onions, cut into thin moons
2 bay leaves
4 tablespoons olive oil
pinch powdered saffron
2 cloves garlic, grated
4 tablespoons chopped parsley
slices of stale bread

Put the garlic in a big pot when the olive oil is hot. When the garlic is almost brown, add the onions, bay leaves, parsley and 1 cup water. Put the mussels in a saucepan, without water; cover and set over low flame until they open. When the mussels are open, some juices will collect in the pot. Save liquid, but try to avoid the sand that may lie on the bottom.

Wash, scale and cut the fish into big pieces. Tie them in a bag of thin cloth. Put the bag into the pot with the mussels, mussel liquid, onions, garlic, etc. and add water so that everything is well covered. Cook for 45 minutes over a high flame. Serve the fish in a separate plate, the soup in a bowl with 2 slices of stale bread.

MINESTRONE INVERNALE
(Winter soup)
(for 6 persons)

> 1/2 cup chick peas
> 3 tablespoons sesame oil
> 1 onion, medium size, minced
> 1 minced stalk celery
> 1/4 head savoy cabbage, shredded
> 2 zucchini, cut into 1-inch strips
> 1 turnip, cut into 1-inch strips
> 1 carrot, minced
> 1 pumpkin, cut into 1-inch strips
> 3/4 teaspoon sea salt
> 5 cups (about) water
> 2 cups brown rice
> 3 teaspoons tamari

Soak chick peas overnight or partially cook them. Drain. Heat oil in soup kettle and sauté vegetables in following order: onion, celery, cabbage, zucchini, turnip and pumpkin. Add salt. Cool the kettle and add the water and chick peas. Simmer for 2 hours, covered, stirring occasionally. Add rice and simmer until rice is done; about 45 minutes. Continue occasional stirring, turning the soup up from the bottom since it is a very thick soup and may have a tendency to stick. Add a little hot water from time to time, if necessary. When soup is done, add **tamari**.

SOUP STOCK

Soup stock is indispensable in Japanese cuisine and is the equivalent of court bouillon in France. Two sorts are common in Japan, one made out of miso paste and one made out of dried fish. Both are widely used, depending on the season and the meal being served. Soup stock serves so many purposes—it even covers up the faults one makes in cooking—you will appreciate having it on hand.

STOCK MADE WITH DRIED BONITO:

Cut 1/4 ounce dried bonito into very thin pieces, thinner than a match. Cut a 2-inch square piece of kombu. Clean the seaweed with a piece of cloth and place into pot with 5 cups water. Add salt and bring to a boil. Remove kombu as water starts boiling. Lower the flame and add the dried pieces of bonito. When water comes to a boil, remove the pan from the fire and let it stand for a few minutes. Usually the bonito settles on the bottom of the pan. Pour the liquid into a strainer. It's ready.

STOCK MADE WITH MISO PASTE:

Bring to a boil 3 or 4 cups water. Add a 2-inch square piece of cleaned kombu. Remove kombu as water starts boiling. Add bonito for 5 minutes, strain. Add a little bit of salt. Add miso paste and let simmer 20 minutes.

About fasting

"How about fasting, Sensei?" asked a student.

The Master looked at the young man, then turning his head to the others, said:

"Fasting is very good for health. It can cure any sickness. But it can also be very dangerous, for the change is so fast that a person can panic and make mistakes."

Fish and seafood

STUFFED MACKEREL

2 1-pound or smaller mackerel
2 onions, grated
2 leeks, grated
2 sprigs parsley, minced
3/4 cup water
1/4 cup tamari
1/4 teaspoon ginger, freshly grated

Use small mackerel, less than 1 pound each. Make sure they are fresh. Use whole fish, viscerated and slit down the middle. Marinate vegetables in water seasoned with tamari and ginger. Let stand for 1 hour, then spoon out vegetables to stuff fish. Put mackerel in baking dish and pour rest of marinade over it. Bake 20 to 30 minutes at 300°. Shut off oven, leaving fish for 5 to 10 minutes. If fish is still too moist, put under broiler for 5 minutes.

SHRIMP CROQUETTES

>10 shrimp, large
>1 egg, separated
>somen (Japanese vermicelli), cut into small pieces.
>2 tablespoons flour
>salt
>pinch thyme powder
>pinch oregano

Shell shrimp. Mash flesh until creamy. Add egg white and white unbleached flour to the mashed shrimp. Add salt, thyme and oregano. Form balls a little smaller than ping-pong balls. Roll in white unbleached flour. Roll in beaten egg yolk and then in somen. Fry in 1/2-inch deep oil for 3 or 5 minutes.

Serve accompanied with nituke or raw watercress and, of course, rice, always rice!

SHRIMP WITH CAULIFLOWER
(for 4 persons)

This great dish turned up in a recipe credited to the Ohsawa Foundation in Chico, California. It is a perfect solution for a dinner party where the guests may be partly macrobiotic and partly full of chemicals. It is a great way to introduce converts into the mysteries of macrobiotic cooking, since almost everybody likes shrimp and the flavor suggests the cuisine at the best Chinese or Japanese restaurants.

> 1 pound shrimp
> 1/2 pound onions, cut in 8 pieces
> 1/2 pound cauliflower, cut in flowerettes
> 4 tablespoons soy sauce
> 2 tablespoons oil
> 2 tablespoons kuzu, diluted in 4 tablespoons water
> 1/4 teaspoon sea salt, or to taste

Peel and devein the shrimp, saving the shells. Dust the shrimp with salt and let them stand. Boil the shrimp shells in 2 cups of salted water for 15 minutes, making a stock. Discard the shells and reserve the stock. Sauté the onions in oil until they begin turning golden. Then add the cauliflower flowerettes and continue to sauté for several minutes. Next, add the stock, cover and let simmer slowly for about 15 minutes until the vegetables are nearly cooked. Slowly add the kuzu diluted in water, stirring all the time. Cook until the simmering sauce becomes transparent and thick. Then add the soy sauce, about 1/4 teaspoon of sea salt, and finally, the shrimp. Cover and boil for 5 minutes, until the shrimp turn pink in the clear brown sauce.

Serve over warm brown rice and be prepared for remarks like: "If *this* is macrobiotics, I think I could interest Irving in it. I really do."

BOILED SARDINES A LA JAPANESE

>12 sardines
>1/4 cup umeboshi juice
>soy sauce, to taste

Take off the heads of a dozen small sardines. Open the bellies, clean. Put the sardines in pan with 1/4 cup umeboshi juice (*see* Sauces). Cover and simmer for 1/2 hour. Then add soy sauce to taste and let simmer again, until liquid is evaporated. Serve hot.

BOILED OYSTERS A LA JAPANESE

>3 doz. oysters
>salt
>5 tablespoons sake
>5 tablespoons tamari
>4 cups soup stock
>3 cups rice

Put oysters in a colander, sprinkle them abundantly with salt and wash them under water. Drain off the water. Put oysters in a large plate and pour on them a mixture of the sake and tamari. Bring to a boil 4 cups of soup stock and add 3 cups of rice. Cook 30 minutes. Add oysters, cover the pot and cook 20 minutes more. Serve with either fresh finely chopped watercress or dandelion sprinkled on the top or served on the side.

MARINATED CRAB IN UMEBOSHI JUICE

    1 crab
    2 stalks celery
    1 cucumber
    salt
    umeboshi juice
    tamari
    oil

Remove stringy parts of celery stalks and cut stalks into 2-inch lengths. Cut again into thin slices lengthwise, soak in water for a few minutes and drain. Boil crab, let cool, take off the shell and shred the meat. Cut a cucumber into thin slices, sprinkle with salt and drain by pressing with hands. Prepare umeboshi juice, mix it with a tiny bit of tamari and vegetable oil. Mix this sauce with celery, cucumber and crab. Serve cool, with cold or hot rice.

If you are not a crab eater use tuna or swordfish as a substitute.

SCALLOPED OYSTERS

    4 tablespoons sesame oil
    3/4 cup brown rice flour
    pinch of saffron
    1 teaspoon sea salt
    4 tablespoons onion, chopped
    1 tablespoon parsley, chopped
    1 clove garlic, small, chopped
    1 tablespoon tamari
    1 quart oysters
    2 cups bread crumbs

Heat oil and slowly stir in the rice flour. Stir over rather high flame until flour starts to darken. Add the saffron and salt, and continue stirring until rice flour is golden. Add onion, parsley and garlic and continue stirring until the rice flour is dark brown, being careful not to burn. Remove pan from heat and stir in the tamari. Poach oysters in their own juice for 2 minutes. Combine oysters and liquor with the vegetable mixture. Pour into baking dish, sprinkle with bread crumbs and bake in a hot oven, 400°, for 30 minutes.

LOBSTER CANTONESE

    2 tablespoons sesame oil
    1 small sliver garlic, minced
    4 scallions, minced
    1 pound lobster meat, cut into 1-inch pieces
    3 tablespoons tamari
    1-1/2 cups boiling water
    1 teaspoon kuzu
    1/4 cup cold water
    1 egg, fertilized, optional

Heat the oil, add the garlic and scallions. Sauté lobster, stirring constantly. Add the tamari and boiling water and mix. Cover and simmer for 10 minutes over a low flame. Dissolve kuzu in cold water and add slowly, stirring until the sauce is thick, smooth and transparent. Turn off the heat. Beat egg lightly and pour over the lobster; stir.

FISH LOAF OR FISH CAKES

        2 cups bread crumbs or cooked rice
        1 cup water
        2 cups boned cooked fish (any white-meat fish)
        2 tablespoons sesame oil
        4 tablespoons whole wheat flour
        1 teaspoon sea salt
        1 egg, fertilized
        1 large scallion or regular onion, chopped
        1 stalk celery, chopped
        2 tablespoons parsley, chopped
        corn oil and sesame oil, combined 1/2 and 1/2, for frying

Soak bread crumbs or rice (bread crumbs are better to use) in water for 1/2 hour. Add the fish, oil, flour and salt. Beat the egg and add, mixing ingredients together by hand. Sauté the scallion, celery and parsley and add, continuing to mix by hand. Form a solid loaf and bake for 3/4 hour in 350° oven. This dish can be served hot or cold. To make fish cakes, mold into hamburger-size patties, dip into whole wheat flour and deep fry in 1/2 sesame oil and 1/2 corn oil. Fish cakes may be baked instead of deep fried.

POLENTA CON VONGLE
(Cornmeal and clams)

polenta: 6 cups water
1-1/2 teaspoons sea salt
2 cups cornmeal
1 tablespoon sesame oil

clams: 1 dozen clams, medium sized
2 tablespoons sesame oil
1 clove garlic, minced
1 pinch oregano
1 tablespoon parsley

Prepare polenta by bringing water to a boil and slowly adding the cornmeal and salt. Stir constantly over low flame for about 10 minutes until smooth, thick and creamy. Then simmer for 30 to 40 minutes. About halfway through the cooking, add 1 tablespoon oil. Shell the clams and chop or cut into pieces, reserving the liquor. In a skillet, heat 2 tablespoons oil with the garlic and oregano. Add chopped clams and simmer for about 2 minutes. Add the parsley and clam liquor and raise flame until liquor is reduced a little. Sauce should not be too liquid. Do not overcook or the clams will be tough. Put hot polenta in soup plates and garnish with clam sauce.

FRESH HERRING IN WHITE WINE
(for 8 persons)

Herring is very yang and wine is very yin. It does not mean that a dish with both is a perfect balance. Wine is less yin when it is aged and is therefore more "willing" to be balanced. Anyway wine here serves only as a sauce. This recipe is perfect for a summer evening, served with cold rice and a little bit of salad.

8 fresh herrings, medium sized
3 glasses white wine
3 glasses water
3 onions, minced
2 tablespoons parsley, chopped
1 bay leaf
1 pinch thyme
salt to taste

Put in a saucepan everything but the fish. Bring to boiling point and cook over low flame for 40 minutes. Clean the herrings—keep the roe, if any—and put them for 10 minutes into the hot sauce. Remove the herrings and let them cool. Boil sauce until half evaporated. Keep the flame low. Remove sauce from fire, cool, and pour on the herrings. Serve cold.

WHITE FISH IN BEAUJOLAIS

Sometimes here and there, as you may have noticed, I have used wine. Why? Simply because I lived in France for 15 years, and what I ate there was so well prepared and so good. Just to make you happy, try it!

>3 pounds white fish
>1 onion, finely chopped
>1 tablespoon parsley
>2 cloves garlic
>5 tablespoons olive oil
>1 tablespoon white unbleached flour
>2 glasses red wine
>salt

Cut the fish into 1-inch pieces and sprinkle with salt. Place on a big plate. Chop finely onion and garlic cloves and sauté them in olive oil in a heavy saucepan. Sprinkle the flour over the oil as you stir. Add 1-1/2 glasses of water and the wine. Add parsley and bay leaf. Simmer for 15 minutes. Add the pieces of fish. Cover the saucepan and allow to cook for another 15 minutes.

FISH BALLS

Only a grandmother should succeed in making a dish like this one. I am not a grandma but I did it!!

> 2 pounds whitefish, ground
> 2 eggs
> 1 cup matzoh meal
> (or 1/3 cup flour)
> 4 tablespoons parsley, chopped
> 1 stalk celery
> 5 tablespoons olive oil
> 2 cloves garlic, crushed
> 1 bay leaf
> pinch thyme
> 2 cups water

Ask the man in the fish market to remove the bones of a whitefish. Ask him also to grind it for you. To the ground fish add the eggs and matzoh meal. If you have no matzoh meal in hand, use 1/3 cup white flour. Add the finely chopped parsley and mix thoroughly. Cut celery, removing strings. Heat 5 tablespoons of olive oil in a large, heavy saucepan and add the crushed garlic, bay leaf and thyme. Put celery on the top of the sauce. Add water and cover. Cook over medium flame 20 minutes. While celery is cooking, make fish balls ping-pong size. Place the balls delicately on the top of the celery. Cook 15 minutes more.

MAMEE FISH

>red snapper
>4 tablespoons olive oil
>2 cloves garlic, crushed
>2 bay leaves
>2 tablespoons parsley, chopped
>pinch thyme
>salt

Clean a red snapper. Cut it into large pieces. Heat olive oil in a heavy saucepan. Add crushed garlic, bay leaves, chopped parsley and thyme. Simmer 2 minutes. Place the pieces of fish in the saucepan. Sprinkle with salt and add 1-1/2 cups water. Cook over medium flame until it comes to a boil. Lower the flame and let simmer 20 minutes.

You can bake the fish in a 350° oven instead of cooking it in a pan. If you wish to do so, do not cut it; it makes a more attractive dish.

SUNO MONO

>2 or 3 stalks celery
>1/4 pound shrimp or crab
>2 cucumbers, medium size
>salt
>raisins

Cut cucumber into thin slices and sprinkle with salt. Let stand 5 or 10 minutes and press with hands to squeeze out the water. Make umeboshi juice (*see* Sauces) and pour it on crab or shrimp and celery cut into small pieces. Garnish with raisins. Serve cold in summer.

BROILED FISH

Almost all kinds of fish can be broiled; it all depends on how you broil them, for how long and with what kind of sauce. However, swordfish, halibut, striped bass, flounder, sole, red snapper, herring, sardines and mackerel are preferable.

Since appearance is important, first broil the side that will be on top when the fish is served. The Japanese place a whole fish with its head to the left, tail to the right and its belly toward the person served. When you broil slices of striped bass, always serve it with the skin side on top.

Courage is of first importance in cooking, so when you broil fish don't be timid and use a low flame; a strong flame is best for this kind of cooking.

Turn over the pieces of fish when browned and broil the other side. Usually the first side takes longer.

A very simple sauce for broiled fish:

> 10 tablespoons soya sauce
> 3 tablespoons water
> 1/2 teaspoon fresh ginger, grated

Mix soya sauce with water. Add grated ginger. Soak fish in the sauce and place it in the broiler. When the first side is browned, turn over and pour on the other side 1 tablespoon of the same sauce and brown.

TERI-YAKI (Japanese Sauce)

> 10 tablespoons soya sauce
> 15 tablespoons rice wine (mirin)

This sauce goes particularly well with fish containing larger amounts of fat. Halibut and swordfish are perfect for teri-yaki. Mix soya sauce with mirin (rice wine). Cook sauce in small saucepan over medium flame. Remove from fire when 1/3 has evaporated. Just before the fish is broiled, pour on it 1 tablespoon of the sauce. Serve the fish as hot as possible.

KOULIBIAC

> 2 slices fresh salmon
> 1/2 pound white unbleached flour
> 2 egg yolks, fresh
> 1 egg, fresh
> 1 egg, hard-boiled
> 2 tablespoons corn oil
> 1 green cabbage, small
> 2 onions, large
> 1 cup fried rice
> 2 tablespoons parsley, chopped
> salt
> 1 cup water

Slice the salmon and boil in water for 10 minutes. Cut salmon into smaller pieces and fry in oil over a high flame. Put aside on a plate. Finely chop hard-boiled egg with parsley. Slice onions into thin moons and sauté lightly. Add the salmon to the chopped egg and parsley. Make a dough by mounding the 1/2 pound of flour and placing an egg yolk in the center, adding corn oil, salt, 1 cup water. Mix and roll dough into a circle less than 1/4 inch thick.

Cover one half of dough circle with 1/4 inch of fried rice, add cabbage leaves that have been soaked in boiling water for 5 or 10 minutes. Place on cabbage alternately the salmon mixture and sautéed onions.

Fold over the other half of the crust, just as you would for a chausson or a piroshki. Press the edges together with a fork and brush the top with egg yolk.

Make a small funnel out of aluminum foil, with the bottom hole 1/2 inch in diameter. Stick it in the center of the top crust. Bake in the oven at 425° for 45 minutes. A few minutes before koulibiac is taken out, pour into the funnel a beaten egg. Return koulibiac to oven for 3 minutes. Remove funnel. Serve hot.

LE COULIS AU HADDOCK
(for 6 persons)

>1 pound haddock filet
>1 pound onions, finely chopped
>1/2 pound carrots
>1/2 pound zucchini
>1/2 red pepper
>pinch thyme
>pinch oregano
>2 bay leaves, small
>7 tablespoons corn oil

Sauté onions in oil over a medium flame for 15 minutes. Cut the vegetables and add them to the onions. Add salt and seasonings. After 15 minutes, lower the flame, cover the saucepan and simmer 15 minutes. Cut the filet of haddock into 6 equal parts and place them on the top of the vegetables. Cover, and simmer again 15 minutes. Serve hot with rice.

CODFISH A LA CATALANE
(for 6 persons)

Fine in summer on the beach.

>1 pound codfish filet
>2 onions, large, minced
>5 garlic cloves
>2 red peppers
>2 leek tops
>pinch thyme
>pinch oregano
>2 bay leaves
>3 tablespoons oil
>2 glasses dry white wine
>sauce bechamel

Boil the cod in water for 10 minutes. Take it out and break up with a fork. Keep the water in which it was boiled. Sauté the onions with leek and garlic cloves in the oil. Brown the mixture in a saucepan and to it add peppers, 1 cup of the fish water, the spices and the wine. Simmer 1/2 hour. Pour half of this mixture into a baking dish. Place the fish in it and cover with the remaining mixture. Pour heavy sauce bechamel on the top and place dish in the broiler or in oven for 15 minutes. Serve hot with rice.

LA QUICHE

La quiche and the crêpe are competing for the title which the quiche lost ten years ago. Both quiche and crêpe come from Brittany, although all kinds of quiches are made in other provinces.

Dough: 1/2 pound pastry flour or half and half whole wheat and unbleached flour
2 tablespoons oil
pinch salt
water, lukewarm

Filling: 12 shrimp
2 eggs
2–3 tablespoons water
salt
tamari

Make a dough by adding lukewarm water to the pastry flour (or whole wheat and unbleached flour, oil, and salt. The dough should be firm. Let it stand at least 1 hour. Then roll the dough into a circle and place it in a round mold. Fry a dozen shrimp in oil, adding tamari, just before removing from pan. Place the shrimp on the crust. Beat the eggs, add 2 or 3 tablespoons of slightly salted water and pour this mixture on the shrimp.

Bake in the oven 20 minutes at 400°. Prepare sauce bechamel. Take the quiche out and pour the bechamel on the top of it. Return to oven for 10 to 15 minutes longer.

In place of the shrimp you can use herring.

HADDOCK A LA CHINOISE
(for 6 persons)

>1 pound haddock
>3 onions, medium size, finely chopped
>6 tablespoons oil
>1-1/2 pints hot water
>5 tablespoons tamari
>15 tablespoons brown rice

Cut the haddock into pieces. Heat the oil in a heavy saucepan and fry the haddock lightly in it. Remove the haddock. In the same saucepan sauté the finely cut onions. Add the rice and keep stirring gently with a wooden spoon. Put the haddock back and add hot water mixed with tamari. Pour hot water until the rice is entirely covered. Cover the saucepan and simmer 40 minutes. Add water if needed.

The wisdom in grains...

Then said Daniel to Melzar, "Prove thy servants, I beseech thee, ten days; and let them give us pulse [grain] to eat, and water to drink. Then let our countenances be looked upon before thee, and the countenance of the children that eat of the portion of the King's meat: and as thou seest, deal with thy servants."

So he consented to them in this matter, and proved them ten days. And at the end of the ten days their countenances appeared fairer and fatter in flesh than all the children which did eat the portion of the King's meat.

Thus Melzar took away the portion of their meat, and the wine that they should drink; and gave them pulse.

As for these four children, God gave them knowledge and skill in all learning and wisdom: and Daniel had understanding in all visions and dreams.

"Main dishes"

PIROSHKI

This is a great Russian and Polish delicacy, usually served hot as an accompaniment to a hearty soup.

Prepare pie crust according to the simple recipe on Page 172. Roll it out and cut into round pieces, 3 or 4 inches across. Take slivered carrots, onions, cabbage, watercress and sauté them in a tiny bit of oil. Then add boiled rice and salt. Form this rice and vegetable mixture into small balls, one for each round of pie crust. Fold over the crust into a half circle, press the edges together with a fork.

These hearty little piroshkis may be fried in deep oil or baked in a 350° oven. If you bake them, brushing beforehand with beaten egg yolk gives them a real professional glaze. Children of all ages enjoy small individual pies.

GYOZA

Gyoza is the Japanese version of Chinese wonton, Jewish kreplach, Italian ravioli.

Add a little salt to whole wheat flour and knead with water to form a soft dough. Keep working the dough until it is soft and has sheen. Roll it out very thin and cut into round pieces 2 or 3 inches across.

Sauté finely diced vegetables such as onion, carrot, watercress, cabbage, seasoning with salt. Add a little flour to the vegetable mixture. Heap small amounts into the rounds of dough. Fold over the dough, keeping the shape long and narrow for even, quick cooking. Seal the edges by pressing with a fork. Drop the gyoza into boiling water and cook until done. Fish them out of the water with a perforated spoon.

Gyoza may be served many ways; in soup like wontons and kreplach, or with a sauce of tamari or miso cream like ravioli. Like wonton, previously boiled gyoza may also be fried in a little oil until crisp, or they may be fried in deep oil.

Even this is not the end of the line. Fried gyoza may be placed in a baking dish, covered with thin rice cream or sauce bechamel and baked.

For entertaining, add shrimp, fish or a little white meat of chicken to the vegetable filling.

GREEN ROAD LINED WITH BROWN AND YELLOW TREES

This recipe is not only good but nice to look at. It is so easy to make, you will not believe it until you have made it. It takes time to make, yet it does not take much room on a plate. You might wonder if making it is worth the candle. But you should not miss presenting such a jewel to your guests.

> 1 cup buckwheat groats, toasted and blended
> 1 cup polenta (Italian cornmeal, available in Italian stores)
> sauce bechamel, made with onions (*see* Sauces)
> macrobiotic bread made of different flours and grains (for 4 servings, 8 slices, 1 by 3 inches long)
> parsley, chopped
> corn oil for frying
> salt
> tamari

Cook the buckwheat like rice cream, with 4 cups of water for 1 cup of buckwheat. Add salt and keep stirring until boiling point. Using another pot, bring water to a boil, add polenta slowly while you keep stirring. Both buckwheat and polenta take 15 minutes to cook after the boiling point is reached. When cooked, place the creams—both of which are very heavy—in separate plates. Better yet, pour each into separate rectangular glass molds. Let stand until jelled. Remove molds and cut polenta and buckwheat puddings into pieces the size of the slices of bread, but a little bit thicker.

Fry both sides of polenta and buckwheat slices in a little bit of corn oil. Pour a mixture of 1/2 tamari and 1/2 water on the slices while they are frying. Heat the bread by frying it the same way.

It is time now to start serving: Place two slices of fried bread side by side less than 1/4 inch apart. Pour 1 tablespoon of hot bechamel sauce on each slice and cover one slice of bread with polenta and the other with buckwheat. Sprinkle the empty space with parsley and serve it as hot as possible, using a teaspoon or a fork as in eating a pie.

HACHIS PARMENTIER

Monsieur Parmentier created a lot of trouble, for it was he who imported the potato to France. First the peasants resented it; their instinct told them it came from hell. How to convince those stubborn and healthy people?

A devilish idea came across the mind of the potato importer; he knew the French were curious and, in their spare time, marauders. He put a fence around his potato field and waited. Soon people came by night, and little by little robbed the gentle "patate". The king was happy, his people were becoming more yin and more obedient. This, I believe, is the best television potato commercial I have ever heard of.

Be reassured, Hachis Parmentier—the "plat de resistance" in French boarding schools—is not made of potatoes, although it tastes almost like it!

> 1 cup buckwheat groats
> 4 cups water
> 1 cup red lentils
> pinch thyme
> 1 or 2 bay leaves
> pinch nutmeg
> salt
> bread, macrobiotic
> sauce bechamel

Toast buckwheat groats, blend in a mixer and cook in salt water. Cook red lentils with thyme, bay leaves and nutmeg. Blend in a vegetable mill. The mixture should be thick and have the same texture as buckwheat cream.

Cover the bottom of a large plate completely with macrobiotic bread made, if possible, with a mixture of flour and grains. Cover the bread evenly with sauce Bechamel. Place a layer of buckwheat cream and on the top of it a layer of blended red lentils. Put in oven 30 minutes and serve hot.

CHOU FARCI

This is the French country version of stuffed cabbage, a staple in Brittany where buckwheat is a principal food. It looks a little complicated, but it's as easy as tearing a leaf off a cabbage.

>6 or 8 cabbage leaves, intact
>2 eggs, fertilized, beaten
>1 cup buckwheat groats
>2 cups water
>1/2 teaspoon salt
>2 tablespoons oil

Stir the uncooked buckwheat grains in the salted water. Beat the eggs. Oil well a heavy, covered iron casserole. Lay a leaf of cabbage on the bottom. Pour a layer of the buckwheat onto the leaf and top it with a layer of beaten egg. Cover with another cabbage leaf, buckwheat and egg until you run out of egg and buckwheat. Make sure a cabbage leaf tops the pile. Cover the casserole and bake in a moderate oven for 1-1/2 hours.

If you are handy, you may be able to turn the casserole upside down onto a platter. If possible, place a platter on top of the casserole, and turn the two over together—as a unit. Lift off the casserole, leaving the chou farci on the platter. Otherwise, cut the chou farci up in the casserole and serve like a hunk of pie. Eat it hot and steaming, seasoned with miso or tamari. This is one of those dishes which stick to your ribs, as the peasants say.

STUFFED PUMPKIN OR ACORN SQUASH

>1/2 teaspoon sesame oil
>1/2 cup onions, diced
>1/2 cup cabbage, finely sliced
>1/4 cup carrot, diced
>3 or 4 shrimp, cut in quarters
>1-1/2 tablespoons sesame oil
>1/2 cup whole wheat flour, sifted
>3/4 cup water
>1 teaspoon tamari
>1 small pumpkin or medium acorn squash
>salt

Heat oil in a deep saucepan; sauté onion, cabbage, carrot and shrimp. Add a dash of salt to bring out the taste of the vegetables. Rub 1 tablespoon sesame oil into whole wheat flour and toast. Set the pan into cold water to cool. Add water and tamari, stir until smooth and add to sautéed vegetables. Do not cook. Cut pumpkin in half, scooping out seeds. Pour uncooked sauce into hollows and brush exposed part of the pumpkin with remaining sesame oil. Preheat oven to 450°. Place stuffed pumpkin onto a slightly oiled, heated pan or casserole and add just enough water on the bottom to prevent burning. Bake for 1 hour or until pumpkin is very tender.

STUFFED SUMMER SQUASH WITH BULGUR

1 cup bulgur wheat
1-1/2 cups water
1/2 teaspoon sea salt
1 summer squash
1 onion, minced
1 teaspoon sesame oil
1 teaspoon fresh mint (if dry, just a pinch)
1 teaspoon fresh basil
1 teaspoon fresh parsley

Pressure-cook the bulgur with water and salt for about 25 minutes or cook in the regular way for 1 hour. Scoop out the squash and chop the pieces with the onion, then sauté. Mix with the cooked bulgur, add seasonings and refill the shells. Brush shells with oil and bake in 300° oven for 45 minutes.

SOBA BUCKWHEAT NOODLES

Make court bouillon (soup stock) with:

> 4 cups of water
> 1 cup tamari
> 1 cup Mirin (rice wine)
> 1/2 ounce dried bonito
> a piece of kombu

Combine liquids, add bonito and kombu. Bring to a boil. Remove from fire and drain through a strainer. Serve this court bouillon in small individual bowls. Also serve on the side in small dishes: minced onions, grated horseradish and crushed nori seaweed, preferably toasted.

Cook soba this way: To boiling water, add soba and salt. When water starts boiling again, add a little bit of cold water to stop the boiling. When it comes to a boil again, drain soba under cold water. Wash until noodles are no longer slimy.

Dip the soba in soup stock, with a fork or chopsticks, and eat, holding the bowl of noodles and hot soup stock as near as possible to your mouth.

NOODLES A LA HUNGARIAN

>3 tablespoons sesame oil
>3 Spanish onions, large, sliced
>4 to 6 scallions, finely chopped
>1 small head cabbage, shredded
>1 package buckwheat (soba), semolina or udon noodles
>1 teaspoon sea salt

In a casserole, sauté in sesame oil the onions, then scallions and then the cabbage. Stir constantly over a medium flame until vegetables are tender. Add a dash of salt. Turn down flame, cover and let vegetables simmer in their own juice for 10 minutes or until lightly browned. Uncover and raise the flame for 1 or 2 minutes so that steam evaporates. Boil noodles with salt until soft; drain. Add to vegetables, mixing thoroughly. Cover and simmer for 5 minutes more. Shut off fire and let stand uncovered (to prevent oversoftening) until ready to serve. Reheat, if necessary, to serve.

ONION PIE

>1-1/2 pounds onions
>dough for 2-crust pie

Sauté onions. Prepare a batch of pie crust. Fill the unbaked pie shell with the sautéed onions. Cover the pie with a top crust and bake for about 1/2 hour in a 350° oven until the crust is golden. Serve hot with chopped parsley on the top.

CARROT OR PUMPKIN PIE

>3 bunches carrots
>or 2 pounds pumpkin
>1 tablespoon sesame oil
>2 onions, sliced
>1 teaspoon sea salt
>1/2 cup water
>1/2 teaspoon cinnamon
>dough for 1 or 2 crust pie

Slice the carrots or pumpkin into large pieces, about 1 inch thick. Heat oil in a pressure cooker and sauté the carrots with the onions. Add the salt and water and pressure-cook slowly for 15 minutes. Cool vegetables, then purée in a blender, ricer or by hand with a fork. In puréeing, use the cooking water and also blend in the cinnamon. For finer texture, puréed vegetables may be strained. Prepare the dough. On a floured board, roll out the dough into 2 crusts to fit a pie plate. Oil the plate lightly and preheat; arrange the purée between the crusts, pie fashion. Brush some sesame oil (or egg yolk) on top and bake in 350° oven for about 1/2 hour.

Instead of covering the pie with a crust, sprinkle the top with Wheatena rubbed with sesame oil to make a crumb pie.

FLAMICHE

> dough for 1-crust pie
> 2 pounds leeks
> sauce bechamel
> oil

Make a dough with half whole wheat and half unbleached flour. Roll out the dough quite thick and large enough to fit a pie plate. Bake the shell for 20 minutes in 375° oven. Sauté leeks in oil, cover the pan and cook 15 to 20 minutes. Take out the crust from the oven. Mix leeks with sauce bechamel, put the mixture into the crust and put back in oven for 10 to 15 minutes.

PIZZA

> whole wheat flour
> white unbleached flour
> yeast powder
> azuki beans
> pinch thyme
> pinch coriander
> bayleaf
> pinch nutmeg

If you have cooked azuki beans, blend them in a vegetable mill or blender. Add thyme, coriander, bayleaf and nutmeg. Mix ingredients well. Flatten the dough with hands on flat metal platter. Pour the brownish mixture delicately on the top of the dough. To make it fancier, add green or black olives and very small pieces of red pepper. Bake in 375° oven for about 1/2 hour.

WHOLE WHEAT QUENELLES

Make a firm dough with whole wheat flour (one egg or two optional). Knead and roll the dough into cigar forms. Cut into 1-inch pieces. Cook 15 minutes in salted boiling water. Serve with sauce bechamel prepared in the usual way, but add to it a tiny bit of garlic powder and one teaspoon of sesame seeds. You can use these cooked quenelles in other ways; for instance, instead of serving them boiled, deep fry them 3 or 4 minutes in oil. Buckwheat flour can be used instead of whole wheat.

WHOLE WHEAT NOODLES

1) Place noodles in salted boiling water and cook over medium flame about 15 minutes. Drain, and serve with nituke.

2) In oil, sauté onions, scallions or leeks, turnip, cabbage and carrots finely cut. Add hot water, add salt. Put noodles in pan with the vegetables, add a pinch of thyme and one bay leaf. When noodles come to a boil, add a tablespoon of chopped parsley. Cook 25 minutes.

3) For a gratinée proceed as for the preceding recipe, adding more water and pumpkin purée. Put in a platter, pour sauce bechamel on the top and bake in 350° oven for 20 minutes.

How about cold drinks?

"One should never drink anything too cold or too hot. Cold water for example is very bad for the intestines—it paralyzes them. It induces pain and causes constipation, and is a source of many sicknesses. In a sense, one should even chew water, for the water is made less cold and is mixed with saliva, which is alkaline."

Gomasio

Sesame salt

Gomasio is our table salt. It is our heartburn remedy . . . if there is heartburn!! It is an indispensable companion in case of seasickness. But only yin people get seasick; if you are yang, you certainly don't need it.

Gomasio is made from sea salt and sesame seeds. The proportion of salt to sesame seeds varies according to condition: *1 part salt to 5 parts sesame seeds* is reasonable.

Toast salt first. Salt should be toasted until it looks crystalline, sparkling. Then grind it in a suribachi, a ridged ceramic bowl with a wooden pestle, very quickly until powdered.

Rinse sesame seeds in a strainer. Toast, stirring constantly over regular flame. They should be evenly browned and, when pinched between fingers, should crumble easily.

Grind sesame seeds and salt together in a suribachi. Handle pestle by holding the top of the stick with the left hand, and the bottom with the right. Grind until the sesame seeds are thoroughly mixed with the salt, and mixture is a powder.

Prepare gomasio weekly, and keep in airtight jar. Do not allow moisture or heat near.

About chewing

The lecture is now over. The Master relaxes in an armchair with a few selected disciples sitting in front of him on the floor. Today, the Master is in a particularly good humor. As he smokes a cigarette, his thought seems very distant yet very near; his disciples wait eagerly to hear and understand it.

At least five minutes pass in the silence of his thinking. Suddenly, a disciple says, "Master, of all the questions that were asked today, there is one that intrigues me more than the others. I would like to know the answer once and for all. What is the image of God, if God made Man in his image?"

"Aha!" says the Master in a low voice; he now adopts the posture of an Indian chief.

All eyes concentrate on the Master's mouth, from which the disciples hope will come the miracle of an answer. The Master, however, lights another cigarette and drags on it. Now a smile comes across his face, furrowing his cheeks, lighting his eyes. The answer comes headlong and without manner:

"Chew, chew very well your food, and you will enter into the kingdom of heaven on earth."

The worst thing

"What is the worst thing a person can do with respect to food?" asked a young man.

The Master didn't hesitate a second before answering:

"It is to eat too much. Overeating leads to many problems, to sicknesses, obesity, and to the most unfortunate thing, no ability to think. Splitting of thought or schizophrenia may occur easily. Man should eat according to his need, not to his pathological hunger for food."

Sauces

A sauce is like a drop of rain on a petal of rose, the morning of a summer day. You can give it any color you want, if the color of the cereal you are serving is dull. A Frenchman would rather die than swallow a dish without setting it off with a sauce. It's his hang-up. It's our delight!

SAUCE BECHAMEL

This basic sauce is very easy to make and very fast.

Heat 1 tablespoon of oil in a saucepan. Add 1 tablespoon of unbleached white flour, stirring to avoid burning. When you get a mixture that is slightly gold-colored, add a cup of lukewarm water. Stir until the sauce is thick. Add salt and, if you wish, ginger, nutmeg or coriander powder, depending on what you are going to use the sauce with. For vegetables, nutmeg is as good as coriander. For broiled swordfish, use ginger.

SAUCE BECHAMEL ONION

This sauce does not take more than 15 minutes to prepare. It's good on rice, buckwheat, and especially on croquettes of any grain.

To 1 pint boiling water, add 2 tablespoons of unbleached flour previously diluted in 1/2 cup water. Add 1 tablespoonful of sesame butter and keep stirring. Add 1 chopped onion, then salt and soy sauce. Cook for 10 minutes. If you wish, add 2 tablespoons of chopped parsley when finished cooking.

SAUCE CUISINIERE UMEBOSHI JUICE

This sauce is very good on any broiled or boiled fish, on salads and on sautéed vegetables, especially dandelion, watercress, spinach, boiled or sautéed lettuce, endives, etc.

Mix together in a bowl: 1 tablespoon of oil, 1 tablespoon of chopped parsley, 1 tablespoon of finely chopped stone leek (Welsh onion), the juice of 3 umeboshi plums and a tiny bit of salt.

Heat a pan and pour into it all ingredients. Cook no more than 2 minutes.

To obtain umeboshi juice, boil 3 salted plums in a cup of water for 5 or 10 minutes. Squeeze them in a strainer by crushing with a fork. This is how the vinegar was made!

SAUCE DES HALLES

Good with chicken or turkey. Must be served on each portion individually.

Chop 4 or 5 shallots and 1 handful of parsley. Put them in a saucepan with 2 cups of water. Add salt and half a roasted pepper. Boil for 30 minutes over a low flame.

SAUCE MAYONNAISE

This sauce is especially good with almost any kind of fish. Its success depends on where you are making it. In a warm room and often in summer, it is very difficult to make. In macrobiotic we do not eat too much fish in summer anyway, it's too yang!

Put an egg yolk in a bowl with a pinch of coriander, salt, and 1 tablespoon of umeboshi juice. While you are mixing, pour in little by little a few drops of olive oil until your sauce is well mixed. A new consistency will tell you when to stop. Add umeboshi juice if necessary.

SAUCE VINAIGRETTE

In a bowl, chop finely half an onion and 2 scallions or shallots. Add 1 tablespoon chopped parsley, 2 tablespoons umeboshi juice, 1 tablespoon soya sauce, 1 tablespoon olive oil and one pinch of coriander powder. Mix thoroughly before serving.

THE LITTLE SAUCE

This sauce is very good on rice and any noodles.

Chop finely 3 medium-size onions, 4 ounces of salsify, 4 ounces of shallots, one handful of chopped parsley, and 2 ounces of anchovies. Cook the mixture in a saucepan 20 minutes over a low flame with 3 tablespoons olive oil and 3 cups water. Remove from the fire and, a few minutes later, add 2 tablespoons of arrowroot. Return to fire and stir until it becomes creamy.

THE GREEN SAUCE

This sauce is perfect for celery, fennel, zucchini, carrots, turnips, etc. It goes also with striped bass, red snapper and fishballs made with whitefish.

Chop a garlic clove finely and sauté it in 2 tablespoons olive oil previously heated in a little saucepan. When the garlic is golden-colored, add a pinch of saffron that has been soaked for a while in 1 cup water. Add 2 tablespoons of finely chopped parsley, salt and 1 cup water. Cook for 15 or 20 minutes.

SAUCE CREVETTE

Chop 1 large clove of garlic finely and sauté it in 2 tablespoons olive oil previously heated in a saucepan. When the garlic is golden-colored, add 4 finely chopped scallions with their green parts. Cook 5 minutes over a low flame. Add a pinch of saffron that has been soaked for a while in a cup of water. Add 3 tablespoons finely chopped parsley and 3 cups water. Simmer. While this mixture is cooking, sauté slightly (not more than 3 minutes) 1 finely chopped onion. To the onion add 4 tablespoons whole wheat flour and 2 cups of water. Stir. The mixture must be heavy. Add parsley and salt.

Now you have two different sauces. Next, boil shelled shrimps in the first sauce you made. Place boiled shrimp on clam shells (3 or 4 in a St. Jacques shell). In a bowl, mix a little bit of each sauce; consistency should be quite thick. Pour this sauce on your shrimps.

You can boil any kind of fish and use it instead of shrimp. Approximate time for preparation: 30 minutes.

PUMPKIN-ONION SAUCE

Serve this sauce with almost all cereals.

Sauté 2 finely cut onions in 1 tablespoon corn oil. Add salt and cook over a very low flame for 20 or 30 minutes. Do the same thing with the pumpkin. In the meantime, prepare sauce bechamel. Add it to the vegetables. Cook for 10 minutes. Mix in a blender with 1 or 2 tablespoons soya sauce.

CHICK PEA SAUCE

Good on rice, millet, etc.

Soak 1 pound of chick peas overnight in warm water. Cut 2 onions and 2 carrots into very thin strips. Sauté them in 1 tablespoon corn oil for 20 minutes. Boil drained chick peas in water. Add the vegetables and cook for 30 minutes. While this is cooking, toast 3 tablespoons of white unbleached flour or semolina. Mix with a little cold water and add to the vegetables. Add salt.

Mix in a blender if you wish to have a creamy sauce.

SAUCE AU GINGEMBRE

Perfect for noodles and buckwheat.

Sauté 3 finely chopped scallions in 1 tablespoon corn oil for 3 to 5 minutes. Add 2 tablespoons sesame butter and 2 tablespoons soya sauce. Add 2 cups water and 1 tablespoon arrowroot previously stirred into 1/2 cup cold water. Add 1/2 teaspoon freshly grated ginger. Simmer 10 minutes. Add salt if needed.

If you want to give this sauce more flavor, add any smoked shellfish or a handful of dashi iriko (small dried fish).

About salt

"According to what you teach one should eat much salt. Do you think it's advisable for everybody?"

The answer came quickly:

"Did I say so?"

"Yes!" answered unanimously the young people around him.

The Master was astonished.

"I am so surprised to hear what you say. Everyone has a different need. You cannot, for example, give the same amount of salt to a child that you can give to an adult. A child is very yang by nature; too much salt will not help him grow. A yin person can take more than others, but with care. If he increases the intake, he may be led to the opposite, become suddenly too yang and lose his ability to judge properly. The change must be very slow. In other words, a yin person must eat in balance and he will become yang naturally. Salt is sometimes a medicine; it must be taken with care. If you don't want to make mistakes, cook with little salt and sprinkle your meals with gomasio. One should avoid being extreme in anything."

Desserts

PIE CRUST

It may be no news to veteran homemakers but, to those who have never attempted pastry before, macrobiotic recipes are simple and easy. Pie dough is not difficult to prepare.

        2 cups whole wheat flour
        2 cups unbleached white flour
        3/4 cup corn oil
        1/2 teaspoon sea salt
        grated orange peel, optional

Mix the flours, salt and grated orange peel, if used, in a large bowl. Mix in the oil with your hands until the dough forms a ball. The secret of a good pie dough is ice-cold water. Add water, mixing with your hands until the dough has a consistency like that of your ear lobe. You will have a better dough if you have not kneaded the flours and water too long. Let stand 1/2 hour before rolling.

The more oil you add the flakier pie crust you will have. You may use ice-cold oil. But then you must roll out the dough immediately.

VARIATIONS

There are several variations of this simple pie crust. You can leave out the orange peel. You can use strong mint tea instead of water to form the dough. You can use whole wheat *pastry* flour mixed with whole wheat flour, or you can use whole wheat pastry flour entirely. If you have not exhausted your quota of 2 tablespoonsful of oil per person per day, you may increase the amount of oil in the pie crust.

AZUKI CHESTNUT PIE

   2 cups azuki beans
   3 cups dried chestnuts
   1 teaspoon sea salt
   cinnamon

Soak the beans and chestnuts overnight in water to cover. Drain.

Pressure-cook them together for at least 1 hour in double the amount of water they were soaked in. Drain off water after cooking. Blend together in an electric blender, using as little water as possible. Season with cinnamon to taste.

Roll out pie crust very thin and bake shell in oven at 400° until brown around the edges. Cool cream and pour into shell. Serve cool with toasted nuts on top (almonds are best).

APPLE PIE

There are several ways to come up with a delicious apple pie. The simplest is the one-crust pie, frosted with kuzu.

>   3 or 4 apples
>   sea salt
>   cinnamon or mint
>   1 tablespoon kuzu
>   5 ounces cold water
>   dough for 1-crust pie

Line a pie plate with pie crust. Slice the raw apples into crescent shapes and arrange them in the shell. Sprinkle the apples with sea salt—a little cinnamon or mint is optional—and bake in a moderate oven until the apples begin to turn brown. Soften the kuzu in an equal amount of cold water, then add it to about 5 ounces of water. Place the mixture over a low flame, stirring it regularly, until it is thick and transparent. Pour the kuzu mixture over the apples and let it cool. If you like the flavor of mint, you may use cooled mint tea instead of water to make the kuzu. For variety you may add a few raisins to the kuzu mixture before pouring it over the pie.

VARIATION

>6 apples, medium size
>1/4 cup apple juice
>Pinch sea salt
>cinnamon to season
>dough for 2-crust pie

In a bowl mix the apple juice and cinnamon. Peel the apples and slice thin into a bowl. Roll out pie crust and line pie plate. Add apples. Heat apple juice and cinnamon mixture with kuzu until thick. Pour over apples. Roll out top pie crust. Cover apples. Seal edges by pressing with fork dipped in water. Bake in oven at 400° until edges are brown, 35 to 45 minutes.

CHESTNUT-APPLE PIE

The chestnut rarely turns up on American menus except as an ingredient for turkey dressing or as marrons glacés, *a sugared topping for ice cream. Perhaps the chestnut is an acquired taste. But it takes very little trying to get to like chestnuts immensely. A good start is to sneak them into an apple pie. They blend with the tartness of the apple to make a solid dessert.*

The ratio of apples to chestnuts should be anywhere from 4 to 1 to 1 to 4. Fresh chestnuts may be slashed and roasted in the oven or in a pan on top of the stove. Or they may be cooked on top of the stove with a salted apple. The chestnut-apple mixture may be put through a vegetable mill. This puree can be used to line a pie plate, with more apples placed on top. It is hard to go wrong. Sometimes the mistakes turn out to be better than what you were aiming for by the book.

This pie works either in a one-crust version, with the apples on top, or in a two-crust version.

Cinnamon, nutmeg, grated orange rind or mint can be used to vary the seasoning. But it is great without any seasoning at all, except the old reliable sea salt.

PUMPKIN OR SQUASH PIE

In the original French version of the Ohsawa book (on which most of these recipes are based) pumpkin pie is listed in the vegetable section. This may mean it is unworthy to be treated as a dessert. This perhaps reflects the French view of the pumpkin. When a Frenchman wants to be insulting about a melon, he denounces it as a "potiron" or pumpkin.

Whatever way you slice it, the pumpkin, or the winter melon, is yang enough to be a winter staple. Some Americans think the Japanese Hokkaido pumpkin—now also cultivated in Europe—tastes more like a squash than what we know as pumpkin.

>1 pumpkin, medium size
>apple juice
>1 egg, separated
>2 tablespoons tahini
>1/2 teaspoon sea salt
>allspice to season
>1 teaspoon vanilla
>oil

Cut pumpkin into small pieces. Sauté in oil. Cover with apple juice, add salt, and cook until soft. Put pumpkin in blender and add egg yolk, tahini, vanilla and seasonings. Blend until it is mixed well. Beat egg white until fluffy. Pour pumpkin mixture into bowl and fold in egg white. Roll out thin pie crust and bake shell in oven at 400° until brown around edges. Pour filling into shell and bake in 350° oven until thick, approximately 15 to 30 minutes.

CHAUSSON

Perhaps it never happens to professional cooks, but beginners usually find they end up with either too much pie crust or too little. If you run short of pie crust, you can always slice what you have into thin strips and make-do with a lattice design. If you end up with too much, make a chausson or two.

Roll pie dough out into thin round pieces, 3 or 4 inches across. Fill half the round with apple butter, apples and chestnuts, or apples and raisins. Fold the other crust half over, just as you would a piroshki, press together with a fork, stick in a moderate oven and bake.

Another trick that will delight the kiddies involves wrapping a layer of thinly rolled pie dough around a clean wooden stick about the size of a man's thumb. Stick it in the oven to bake. When it cools, it may be filled with chestnut puree and served covered with a mixture of coffee substitute and apple butter. Baked squash is also very delicious.

If you want to make a batch of these pastry cylinders in a hurry, deep fry them in oil.

CHAUSSON AUX FRUITS

Prepare pie dough with only pastry flour. Roll out and cut into circles 7 inches in diameter. On one half of a circle spread thick apple sauce and a few raisins. Fold dough over and press edges with a fork. Brush with egg yolk. Bake in oven at 375° for 30 minutes.

SAUTÉED APPLE FILLING

Peel and cut into very thin slices 2 apples. Sauté in 1 teaspoon oil. Add raisins and sliced almonds. Sauté until soft. This filling is good for chausson, individual pies and crêpes.

APPLESAUCE

Applesauce or apple butter make a scrumptious dessert when rolled or folded inside a quartered crêpe. Find some small red flavorful cooking apples, wash them and cut them up, skins and all. Cook in a saucepan with just enough water to keep them from burning. Strain them through a food mill—that will take care of the skins. If you add a few flakes of fresh or dried mint, it gives them a special zip. Or use cinnamon.

If you have a pressure cooker, the whole process takes a fast 5 minutes. Mashed or boiled, or roasted whole, chestnuts can be added to applesauce to change the dish entirely.

APPLE BUTTER

Some health food shops stock a dietetic brand of apple butter made of nothing but apples—no sugar or other additives. It is a handy thing to have in the kitchen—but grandmother made it herself out of applesauce placed in a large heavy pan and cooked slowly on a low, low flame for 3 or 4 hours or so until it was dark brown. This method takes careful watching to keep the applesauce from burning.

FRUIT PIE

>   1 cup semolina
>   4 cups water
>   1/4 teaspoon salt
>   vanilla to season
>   1 cup fruit in season: cherries, strawberries, apples, apricots (be careful—they are very yin!)

Cook semolina with salt and vanilla until thick. Roll out thin pie crust. Add cooked semolina 1/5 inch thick and place fruit evenly on top. Bake in oven at 375° for 30 to 40 minutes. Cook apple juice with water and kuzu until thick. Pour over top of pie. Water may be used instead of, or mixed with, apple juice. Serve cool.

APPLE STRUDEL

Roll out pie dough in a large rectangle to 1/8-inch thickness. On it spread tahini mixed with an equal amount of water. On top of this place an even layer of sliced apples, roasted and crushed almonds, raisins, grated orange peel. Sprinkle with vanilla powder. Fold the rectangle three times as if you were folding paper to put in an envelope. Pinch edges closed with a fork. Brush top with egg yolk diluted with 1 teaspoon of water. Bake in oven at 375° for 45 minutes.

APPLE CRUNCH

Peel and slice thin 10 apples. Place in a baking dish 2 inches deep. Pour on top 1/2 cup apple juice mixed with cinnamon. In a bowl mix together 1 cup whole wheat flour, 1 cup unbleached white flour, 1/2 teaspoon salt, 1/2 cup oil. Mix well and add 1/3 cup apple juice. Work all the ingredients together until the mixture is crumbly. Sprinkle over apples and let stand 1/2 hour. Bake in oven at 400° until apples are soft and juicy and top is beginning to brown.

APPLE DELIGHT

Peel and slice 5 apples into quarters. Bring to a boil 1 cup of water, add 2 tablespoons raisins, a drop of vanilla and grated lemon rind. Then add apples. Cover and cook for 10 minutes over a high flame. Do not break apples. Served cool this is most delicious.

CHESTNUT CREAM

Cook 1 pound of chestnuts in a pot with double amount of water until soft. Drain and blend in an electric blender, using as little water as possible until creamy. Add a pinch of salt and cinnamon to taste. Serve cool with toasted crushed almonds.

CUSTARD

Blend in an electric blender 2 tablespoons tahini and 2 cups water. Place this in a pot with 3 cups apple juice, pinch of salt. Dissolve 3 tablespoons kuzu or arrowroot in a small amount of water in a small bowl. Add this and 1/2 teaspoon vanilla and grated lemon peel to the pot. Cook over medium flame, stirring constantly until thick. Cook for a few minutes and turn into a dish rinsed with cold water. Cool and serve with toasted crushed almonds. This is too good to be yang!

CHERRY PUDDING

Mix cooked rice with pitted cherries boiled in apple juice. Add a pinch of salt and 1/4 teaspoon vanilla. Add bechamel sauce, 1/3 volume of rice. Bake in oven at 350° for 1/2 hour. Serve cool.

APPLE FRITTERS

Mix 1/2 pound of whole wheat pastry flour, 3 large apples peeled and chopped into small pieces, 2 handfuls of raisins and 1/4 teaspoon salt. Add 1 egg. Add water until batter is elastic and light. Drop by tablespoons into 1/2 inch hot oil. Fry until light and slightly browned. These fritters may also be baked.

BUCKWHEAT APPLE FRITTERS

       1 cup buckwheat flour
       1 cup pastry flour
       3 tablespoons corn oil
       1/4 teaspoon sea salt
       1 egg
       1 handful raisins
       cinnamon

Mix well. Dropping by tablespoons, deep fry in oil until light and slightly brown.

PUDDING DE PAIN
(Bread Pudding)

In French the word for pudding is pudding. At the Guen Mai Macrobiotic restaurant on Rue de l'Abbaye in Paris, smack behind the Church of Saint Germain des Pres, they serve a delicious bread pudding. In macrobiotic restaurants, as elsewhere, waste is counted among the seven deadly sins. Tired bread can be salvaged and served with all its food value, salvaged if not enhanced, using the simple tricks they use at Guen Mai.

>   stale bread
>   mint tea or mu tea
>   grated orange rind
>   raisins, nuts, chopped apple
>   cinnamon
>   oil
>   egg, fertilized (optional)
>   salt
>   flour

Slice or chop the stale bread into small pieces and soak it well in mint tea. If you're not wild for mint, try mu tea. Add the grated orange rind, raisins, a few chopped nuts, a finely chopped apple, cinnamon and a tablespoon of oil. Let the mixture marinate for a good hour or two until the flavors have intermingled. Beat the egg well and add it to the mixture, which should have the consistency of a soft dough. If it seems too liquid and runny, add a little whole wheat flour. Almost any cooked cereal may be added as well to give it body.

Heat a bread pan and oil it lightly, then dust it with a fine coating of flour. Pour in the mixture and bake in a medium oven until it pulls away from the sides of the pan.

Bread pudding can be served hot the first time round, but it keeps well for days.

BEIGNETS DE POMME

Here is a simple, speedy and delicious dessert that is served to perfection at the tiny ZEN Restaurant in the courtyard at 40, Rue du Faubourg Montmartre in Paris. "Beignet" in French means the same thing as "tempura" in Japanese.

>   apples
>   salt
>   flour
>   water
>   oil

Core an apple or two, depending on how many guests there are for dinner. One apple for two persons is a generous serving. Whether you peel them is optional. Slice them laterally so you end up with doughnut shaped slices about $1/5$ inch thick. Dust the apples with sea salt or let them cool in a solution of cold salted water.

Make a tempura batter with whole wheat flour or a mixture of whole wheat and unbleached white flours. Shake the apple slices in a small sack with a little whole wheat flour to give them a slight dusting. This causes the tempura batter to adhere and cover the apples completely.

Heat your vegetable oil to $350°$ or a little more. Usually a 3-inch thickness of hot oil is recommended, but with thinly sliced apples you can get by with less. Dip the cooled, salted, flour-dusted apples in the tempura batter and slip them into the hot oil. When they float to the top and brown on one side, turn them over. Drain on paper toweling and serve hot.

For an added fillip, use cooled mint tea instead of water to make your tempura batter.

BAKED APPLE

The old folk saying about an apple a day keeping the doctor away is merely another way of saying that the apple is the most yang of all fruits. Baking apples rids them of excess liquid, making them even more yang. So the baked apple—with or without a pie-crust overcoat—is a staple dessert in the macrobiotic regime. The smaller and redder the apples, the better. A tired-looking cooking apple is apt to produce better results than its shining gorgeous cousin covered with cellophane and full of chemicals.

Remove the core from the apple, from the top—where the stem is, taking care not to pierce the bottom. Remove the seeds and core. Fill the apple with either:

- A mixture of tahini, sesame butter and salt
- Dried raisins
- A mixture of salt and mint leaves, dried or fresh
or • A mixture of grated orange rind and cinnamon

Then bake in a medium oven for 30 or 40 minutes until done.

Even more yang is the baked apple with an overcoat made of pie crust. Prepare apples exactly the same way and place them on a round of pie dough rolled out thin. Wrap the dough around the apple, pinch the top to close it, brush with beaten egg yolk to give it that real bakery-window glaze, and bake in a moderate oven for about 1/2 hour.

One school of thought recommends leaving a tiny opening in the top of the overcoat for the steam to escape. Experiment!

CHESTNUT CROQUETTES

Marie-Antoine Careme is often called one of the greatest chefs of all time. When he was only 17, he was snagged by the wily Talleyrand who knew that the way to a diplomat's pouch was sometimes through his paunch and made strategic use of the state dinner to soften up visiting plenipotentiaries. Careme's first cookbook, Le Patissier Royal, *appeared in 1815 and included, besides pastries,* entremets *or entre-acts, breath-catchers between main courses. One of his entremets made a classic use of the chestnut. By substituting oil for butter and kohkoh for cream, it becomes a deluxe macrobiotic dessert, for the chestnut, next to the apple, is the most yang of all fruits.*

4 (per serving) chestnuts
2 tablespoons oil
2 tablespoons kohkoh, thick and liquefied
2 eggs, fertilized

Roast the chestnuts the way the French street vendors do, by gashing the round side with a sharp knife before putting them in pan or oven. Or, if you wish, they may be boiled. In any case they should be cooked until they are soft and easy to peel. Reserve half the chestnuts whole and mash the other half to give 2 cups loosely packed. Prepare a puree by adding the liquid kohkoh, oil, beaten eggs and salt. Spread the puree on a lightly oiled plate until it is cool enough to mold.

Wrap each whole chestnut in a thick coating of puree. Then dip into beaten egg. Next roll in kohkoh powder (or rice cream or bread crumbs). Fry in deep oil as you would tempura. Or in an oiled baking dish bake in a hot (450°) oven until they are browned on all sides.

Two of these hot wrapped chestnuts make a scrumptious dessert for a special occasion.

APPLE-PUMPKIN DESSERT CREAM

Peel equal amounts of apple and pumpkin. Sauté in a heavy pot for 15 minutes in 2 tablespoons corn oil. Add 1/2 cup water and cook 20 minutes. Add cinnamon, nutmeg and a pinch of salt. Pour into demitasse cups rinsed with cool water. Serve cool with toasted crushed almonds.

CREAM OF FRUIT

Roast 1 cup of oat flakes in 2 teaspoons sesame oil. Let cool. Mix with 3 cups cold water, a pinch of salt. Cook over high flame, stirring constantly, until it boils. Add chopped raisins, 1 plum, 1 apricot, 2 or 3 slices of orange, grated orange peel. Cook 1/2 hour over low flame. Serve cool.

COFFEE JELLO

>2 cups apple juice
>2 cups water
>2 tablespoons Pero or (preferably) dandelion coffee
>1/4 teaspoon sea salt
>handful raisins
>1/2 teaspoon vanilla or grated orange peel

Boil ingredients for 10 minutes. Dilute 2 tablespoons arrowroot in 1/4 cup water and stir in. Cook until thick, stirring constantly. Serve hot or cold with roasted crushed almonds.

HALVAH

Roast 1 cup semolina or cornmeal in 2 teaspoons sesame oil. To 5 cups boiling water add 1/4 teaspoon salt. Stir in flour. Stir constantly until it boils. Add a handful of raisins, 2 peeled apples sliced very thin and cinnamon to taste. Cook 1/2 hour. Turn into dish 2 inches thick, rinsed with cold water. Serve cold with roasted crushed almonds and applesauce.

CLAUDE'S CAKE

       1 cup whole wheat flour
       1/2 cup buckwheat flour
       1/2 cup chestnut flour
       1/2 cup unbleached white flour
       1/2 cup soy flour
       1/2 teaspoon sea salt
       2 tablespoons oil
       1 tablespoon tahini
       apple juice and water, 1/2 and 1/2
       1 teaspoon self-rising yeast
       1 egg
       6 tablespoons raisins
       pinch of cinnamon
       grated orange peel

Mix flours. Add salt and work oil and tahini into flours until evenly distributed. Let stand 20 minutes. Mix 1 teaspoon self-rising yeast with 1/4 cup hot water. Work well into flours. Mix in 1 egg and grated orange peel. Add a handful of raisins. Mix all ingredients with 1/2 apple juice, 1/2 water, until wet and elastic. Flour dough and place in a greased pan. Let stand overnight and bake in oven at 375° for approximately 1-1/2 hours.

Little things to know

Cooked vegetable protein is more yin than animal protein, but becomes more yang than animal protein within the body.

Too much *salt* causes constipation and pain. Too much *liquid* does so also.

Body odor, especially under the arms, comes from animal food. This kind of smell is developed only in animals.

Heartburn: Excessive acidity (yin).

Vitamins: Man started to lose his ability to manufacture them within his body when he started eating too much fruit. This ability changes daily according to our way of eating.

A person in good health should be very sensitive. In the United States 9 out of 10 are not *ticklish* to a light touch.

The *balance* of our foods should not resemble a scale but rather a potential spiral. One should eat according to one's need and keep changing.

Protein is a very bad conductor of *vibrations* coming from infinite expansion. A slim man is a better thinker: *Don Quixote*.

Rice is starchy but its outer layers have the elements necessary to digest *starch*.

Chinese medicine says:
  Bad intestines cause nervousness.
  Bad liver, pancreas, spleen . . . anger, irritation.
  Bad heart, blood circulation . . . anxiety.
  Bad lungs, breathing. . . melancholy.
  Bad nervous system . . . suspiciousness, exclusiveness, skepticism.

There are 5 causes of *obesity:* protein, starch, sugar, fat and water. You can get rid of water very fast but not of fat.

How to test a *dyed tea:* Put the bag of tea in hot water. Dip in a handkerchief. If the tea has been dyed, the cloth will be stained.

A *cramp* is due to excess acid.

A *sneeze, cough, hiccup* are normal reactions of the body to discharge yin.

Itching comes from excess yin.

Whistling is also a reaction to discharge yin. People who whistle are generally milk, chocolate, candy and fruit eaters.

The traditional Japanese *bow* is flexible like a plant in a field. In the West we shake hands: we are meat eaters.

Crying: also expulsion of yin (tears).

When the *feet* are pointed out in walking, it means that the main food of the person is animal food. Pointed in: vegetables.

Blinking is also due to too much liquid (yin). Eyes are desperately trying to expel the excess.

Pimples: extreme yin.

Horizontal lines on the *forehead* are from too much water (yin). Vertical: yang.

Children need less salt and more liquid.

Short-sightedness is from animal foods. *Far-sightedness* is from vegetables and fruits.

Overeating is the biggest enemy of man.

Chewing mobilizes all the muscles of the body.

Breathing is essential. To maintain good health one should breathe deeply from the area of the intestines.

In England the number of cases of stomach *ulcers* dropped during the war but rose again after the war with the return of rich foods.

Appetite is the expression of our body to survive. Pathologic appetite is the desire for only ice cream, for example.

In Spain, they say of an attractive woman *"Que salada!"* (How salty). In the United States we say: "How sweet!!!"

Men who like too many sweets cannot love women. Sweets kill *sexual desire*.

For an increase in sexual desire:
Ginseng works fast. Burdock works over a long period, is considered the best. Fish, especially anchovies, and eggs and buckwheat are good for endurance.

For a decrease in sexual desire:
Dairy foods, soybean products, mushrooms, uncooked seaweed, bamboo shoots, eggplant, potato, raw radish, raw grain.

Frigidity and impotence are fostered by:
Yin fruits such as avocado, papaya, pineapple, etc. Sugar, saccharine. Cold drinks.

Something happened in Paris! The Russian handball team came to Paris with the firm intention of winning the title. As soon as they arrived they went to a restaurant and asked for buckwheat. The restaurant had no buckwheat. So they went to other restaurants and again they were told that there was no buckwheat. Their coach did not hesitate; he simply decided that he and his comrades should fly back to Moscow, and that's exactly what they did. How could a Russian sportsman possibly play without his precious kasha?

It is better to eat foods that are farther back in *biological history*. They widen the scope of thinking, which means good memory.

Raw-food eaters are very much influenced by the forces of nature. Their sexual desire occurs mainly in the spring.

Fire and salt made man more independent, smaller and less passive.

Mixed diet causes *mixed thinking*.

Dandruff is overproduction of skin (too much protein).

Suppression of desire is one cause of schizophrenia. If we try to suppress desire in children, we create *mental illness*. Desire is the motor of growth.

We eat mostly because of *habit;* we do not really have appetite.

Bibliography

Food Is Your Best Medicine, by Henry Bieler (Random House).
You Are All Sanpaku, by George Ohsawa and William Dufty (University Books).
Zen Macrobiotics, The Art of Longevity and Rejuvenation, by George Ohsawa (Ignoramus Press).
The Philosophy of Oriental Medicine, by George Ohsawa (Vol. 1) (Ignoramus Press).
The Book of Judgment, by George Ohsawa (Ignoramus Press).
Zen Cookery, Vol. 1, a treasury of over 400 recipes (Ignoramus Press).
Transmutations biologiques, by Louis Kervran (Librairie Maloine).
A la decouverte des transmutations biologiques, by Louis Kervran (Le courrier du Livre).

The Yellow Emperor's Classic of Internal Medicine (University of California Press).
The I-Ching or Book of Changes, Bollingen Series XIX (Pantheon Books).
Chinese Folk Medicine, by Wallnöfer and Rottausher (Crown Publishers).
The Poisons in Your Food, by William Longgood (Grove Press).

Monthly publications

Yin-Yang, Centre International Ignoramus, 26 Rue Lamartine, Paris 9°, France.
The Macro-Biotic Monthly, Ignoramus Press, Los Angeles, Calif.
The Order of the Universe, Order of Universe Publications, Box 203, Prudential Center Station, Boston, Mass.

Glossary

Aduki
  or azuki beans   Hard red beans from northern Japan.

Bancha   Japanese green leaf tea. Is used as the everyday tea and is quite commonly used in Japan. With a dash of tamari, it gives a very bracing lift to the fatigued.

Bonito flakes   After the bones of the bonito are removed, the fish is cut and dried in drying ovens. The finished product is shaved and used for flavoring. Commonly used Japanese product.

Brown rice   Unrefined rice. Recommended variety is organic, short-grained and carefully milled. The outer coat or gami should not be broken or badly scratched. Should not

	be kept longer than 3 months after picking. Use as soon after purchasing as possible.
Bulgur	A Near Eastern type of semolina or processed wheat.
Burdock	A common but little used wild root vegetable; resembles tree roots.
Cellophane noodles	Chinese noodles, very thin and transparent, made of mung bean.
Chapati	Indian-style flat bread made from any grain or a grain combination and prepared by baking, frying or, most often, holding over fire.
Couscous	Precooked Moroccan-style bulgur.
Daikon	Dried white Japanese radish.
Ginseng tea	Made from the root of the ginseng plant, is used widely as a medicine. Plant grows in the eastern United States as well as other places.
Gomasio	Table seasoning made from ground toasted sesame seeds and sea salt in proportions varying with the season and general activity level. Easily becomes stale and should be prepared weekly (see recipe) and stored in a tightly sealed jar.
Hiziki	Spindle-shaped, small, black seaweed.
Japanese knife	A very sharp, rectangular-shaped steel knife used primarily to cut vegetables. When properly handled, can produce machinelike precision and speed.

Glossary

Kasha	Coarse, cracked buckwheat, millet or barley; commonly buckwheat.
Kokkoh	A blend of cereals and seeds ground into a flour. Used principally as milklike gruel for babies after nursing period.
Kuzu	Vegetable root gelatin from Japan. Used as one would use arrowroot or corn starch.
Lotus tea or Kohren tea	Made from lotus root and raw ginger.
Miso	Japanese soybean paste made by fermenting soybeans with whole wheat and sea salt over a period of 3 years. Is used widely in Japan for miso soup. Commercial preparations are not recommended; only the macrobiotic stores have the right kind.
Mu tea	A very yang beverage from Japan. An herb tea made of ginseng and 15 medicinal plants.
Nituke	Vegetables sautéed.
Nori	Laver or sloke, a kind of seaweed.
Sea salt	Common salt made by the evaporation of sea water with nothing added.
Semolina	Flour or middlings made from the hardest portions of wheat, which resist millstone grinding when whole wheat is stoneground to flour. All spaghetti products once were made from pure semolina.
Soba	Japanese buckwheat noodles. Boiled and eaten with dashi, court bouillon, clear soup stock, etc.

Soy or soya sauce	*See* Tamari.
Suribachi	An earthenware mortar with a wooden pestle, used for grinding sesame seeds and sea salt into gomasio.
Tahini	A Near Eastern product of hulled sesame seeds in the form of a paste. Also called sesame butter.
Tamari	A pure soy sauce concentrate, a byproduct of miso. Commercial soy sauce is not recommended; macrobiotic stores have the right kind.
Tempura	A widely known and much enjoyed Japanese dish of deep-fried fish and/or vegetables.
Tofu	A curd made of the liquid in which crushed soybeans have been softened; it is solidified by boiling.
Udon	A kind of vermicelli similar to soba, but made of cornmeal. A Japanese product.
Umeboshi plums	Plums preserved in salt for 3 years. In Japan, some conservative families still prepare some every year.
Vegetable brush or tawashi	A Japanese brush used for cleaning vegetables.
Wok	Chinese frying pan resembling a salad bowl. Comes in various sizes and is made of iron or stainless steel. The Chinese cook uses his wok for everything, from stir frying to braising to stewing to deep frying.

Recipe index

Aduki Rice, 36
Apple Butter, 179
Apple Crunch, 181
Apple Delight, 181
Apple Fritters, 182
Apple Pie, 174–75
Apple-Pumpkin Dessert Cream, 188
Applesauce, 179
Apple Strudel, 180
Azuki Chestnut Pie, 173
Azuki Soup, 113

Baked Apple, 186
Barley Soup, 98
Beignets de Pomme, 185
La Belle Jardiniere, 108
Boiled Oysters a la Japanese, 130
Boiled Sardines a la Japanese, 130
La Bouillabaisse, 123
Bread, Unyeasted, 53
Bread, Yeasted, 52
Breadsticks, 55
Broccoli (Nituke), 61
Broccoli (Tempura), 71

Broiled Fish, 140
Brown Rice Croquettes, 38
Buckwheat Apple Fritters, 183
Buckwheat Chips, 84
Buckwheat Croquettes, 43
Burdock (Nituke), 61
Burdock Root (Tempura), 70

Cabbage Soup, 117
Carrot Pie, 158
Carrot Roots (Tempura), 70
Carrot Sesame (Nituke), 60
Carrot Soup, 102
Carrot Tops (Tempura), 70
Cauliflower (Tempura), 70
Cauliflower Soup, 114
Caviar of the Poor, the, 81
Celery (Nituke), 61
Celery (Tempura), 71
Chapati, 55
Chausson aux Fruits, 178
Cherry Pudding, 182
Chestnut-Apple Pie, 175
Chestnut Cream, 181

Chestnut Croquettes, 187
Chestnut Rice, 39
Chestnuts (Tempura), 71
Chick Pea Sauce, 170
Chinese Soup, 103
Chou Farci, 153
Clams (Tempura), 72
Claude's Cake, 190
Clear River, 100
Codfish a la Catalane, 144
Coffee Jello, 189
Corn (Tempura), 71
Cornmeal and Clams, 135
Le Coulis au Haddock, 143
Couscous, 45–47
Couscous Rice, 39
Cream of Fruit, 188
Crêpe de Sarasin, 49
Crêpes, 47–49
Cresson sur Canape, 83
Croquettes de Lentilles, 80
Croquettes of Chick Peas, 81
Custard, 182

Dandelion Nituke, 60

Eggs (Tempura), 72
Endive (Nituke), 61
Endives on the Beach, 88

Fish (Tempura), 73
Fish Balls, 138
Fish Cakes, 134
Fish Kebbab (Tempura), 76
Fish Loaf, 134
Fish-Roe Spread, 81
Flamiche, 159
French Onion Soup, 120
Fresh Corn on a Green Field, 105
Fresh Herring in White Wine, 136
Fried Couscous, 47
Fried Kasha, 44
Fried Rice for Guests, 38
Fried Rice with Scallions, 37
Frites, 84
Fruit Pie, 180

Garden Rice Soup, 96
Gomasio, 162
Gomuku Rice, 37
Gratin de Millet, 51

Green Road Lined with Brown and Yellow Trees, 150
The Green Sauce, 168
Gyoza, 149

Hachis Parmentier, 152
Haddock a la Chinoise, 146
Halvah, 189
Hiziki, 65
Hiziki with Lotus or Carrots, 66

Karinto, 85
Kasha Noodles Gratinee, 44
Kasha Varnitchkes, 44
Kasha with Vegetable Gravy, 42
Koi-Koku, 111
Koulibiac, 141

Leaf Vegetables (Nituke), 64
The Little Sauce, 168
Lobster Cantonese, 133
Lotus Root (Tempura), 73

Mamee Fish, 139
Marinated Crab in Umeboshi Juice, 131
Middle Eastern *Meze*, 82
Millet Soup, 107
Millet Vegetable Stew, 50
Minestrone Invernale, 124
Miso in Green, 87
Miso-Onion Spread, 87
Miso Soup, 99
Miso Spread, 86
Mussel Soup, 116

Nituke, 57–64
Noodles a la Hungarian, 157
Nori, 67

Onion Pie, 157
Onions (Nituke), 62
Onions (Tempura), 73
Onion Soup, 119
Oysters (Tempura), 74

Parsnips (Nituke), 62
Parsnips (Tempura), 74
Pie Crust, 172–73

Piroshki, 148
Pizza, 159
Polenta con Vongle, 135
Polenta Soup, 106
Potiron-Pois Chiche, 109
Pudding de Pain, 184
Pumpkin and Bean Soup, 118
Pumpkin-Chick Peas, 109
Pumpkin-Onion Sauce, 169
Pumpkin Pie, 158, 177
Pumpkins (Tempura), 74
Pumpkin Soup, 93–95
Purée de Lentilles, 80
Puréed Turnip Soup, 121

La Quiche, 145

Rice, 36, 77
Rice Balls, 40
Rice Cream, 40
Rice Pie, 41

Sakura Rice, 36
Salade D'Endives, 89
Sauce au Gingembre, 170
Sauce Bechamel, 165
Sauce Bechamel Onion, 166
Sauce Crevette, 169
Sauce Cuisiniere Umeboshi Juice, 166
Sauce des Halles, 167
Sauce Mayonnaise, 167
Sauce Vinaigrette, 168
Sautéed Apple Filling, 179
Scallion Soup, 104
Scalloped Oysters, 132
Scallops (Tempura), 74
Semoulinette, 97
Sesame Rice, 39
Sesame Salt, 162
Shrimp (Tempura), 75
Shrimp Croquettes, 128
Shrimp with Cauliflower, 129
Soba Buckwheat Noodles, 156
Soupe aux Choux, 117

Soupe aux Lentilles, 110
La Soupe de Provence, 122
Soupe Quartier Latin, 117
Soup of Fresh Noodles, 115
Soup of Oat Flakes, 96
Soup Stock, 125
Spread of Sardines, 88
Squash Pie, 177
Stock Made with Dried Bonito, 125
Stock Made with Miso Paste, 125
String Beans (Nituke), 63
Stuffed Mackerel, 127
Stuffed Onion with Millet, 51
Stuffed Pumpkin or Acorn Squash, 154
Stuffed Summer Squash with Bulgur, 155
Summertime, 89
Suno Mono, 139

Tempura, 67–76
(Tempura) Basic Batter, 69
Teri-Yaki, 141
Three Vegetables Nituke, 64
Turnips (Nituke), 63
Turnips (Tempura), 75

Unyeasted Bread, 53

Vegetable Pâté, 78–79
Vermicelli Soup, 101

Wakame, 66
Watercress (Nituke), 63
Watercress (Tempura), 75
Watercress Soup, 100
White Fish in Beaujolais, 137
Whole Wheat Noodles, 160
Whole Wheat Quenelles, 160

Yeasted Bread, 52

Zucchini (Tempura), 76